Basic and Clinical Aspects of Neuroscience Vol. 5

Edited by C. Weil (Managing Editor)
E. E. Müller and M. O. Thorner

O. Lindvall (Ed.)

Restoration of Brain Function by Tissue Transplantation

With Contributions by

O. Lindvall   P. Brundin   A. Björklund   K. Wictorin
S. B. Dunnett   J. Bengzon   F. H. Gage   L. J. Fisher   H. Widner

With 42 Figures and 1 Table

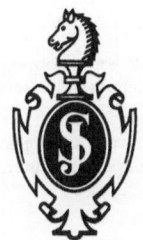
Springer-Verlag
Berlin Heidelberg New York
London Paris Tokyo
Hong Kong Barcelona
Budapest

Dr. Claude Weil
Sandoz Pharma Ltd
4002 Basel, Switzerland

Professor Dr. Eugenio E. Müller
Dipartimento di Farmacologia
Facoltà di Medicina e Chirurgia
Università degli Studi di Milano
Via Vanvitelli, 32
20129 Milan, Italy

Professor Dr. M. O. Thorner
Dept. of Internal Medicine
School of Medicine
University of Virginia
Charlottesville
Virginia 22908, USA

Dr. Olle Lindvall
Restorative Neurology Unit (RNU)
Department of Neurology
University Hospital
221 85 Lund, Sweden

Cover picture: Schematic illustration of selected serial sections at different rostrocaudal levels within the same animal, showing the noradrenergic innervation produced by a seizure-suppressant graft of fetal locus ceruleus tissue in the hippocampus rendered hyperexcitable by denervation.

Volume 1: The Dopaminergic System
© Springer-Verlag Berlin Heidelberg 1985

Volume 2: Transmitter Molecules in the Brain
© Springer-Verlag Berlin Heidelberg 1987

Volume 3: The Role of Brain Dopamine
© Springer-Verlag Berlin Heidelberg 1989

Volume 4: Somatostatin
© Springer-Verlag Berlin Heidelberg 1992

ISBN-13:978-3-540-55823-1   e-ISBN-13:978-3-642-77718-9
DOI: 10.1007/978-3-642-77718-9

Library of Congress Cataloging-in-Publication Data
Restoration of brain function by tissue transplantation / [edited by] O. Lindvall, with contributions by O. Lindvall . . . [et al.]
   (Basic and clinical aspects of neuroscience ; vol. 5)
Includes bibliographical references and index.
   ISBN-13:978-3-540-55823-1

1. Intracerebral transplantation. 2. Fetal nerve tissue – Transplantation. 3. Brain – Diseases – Treatment. I. Lindvall, Olle. II. Series.
[DNLM: 1. Brain Diseases – rehabilitation. 2. Brain Diseases – surgery. 3. Brain Tissue Transplantation. W1 BA813S v. 5 /WL 368 R436] RD594. 12.R47 1993 617.4'81059 – dc20 DNLM/DLC

21/3145-5 4 3 2 1 0 – Printed on acid-free paper

Preface

The first valid attempts at restoring brain function by intracerebral grafting (ICG) were made in 1979 in rats with experimental parkinsonism, and only a few years elapsed before the technique was used as a therapeutic approach in patients with Parkinson's disease (PD). Despite encouraging results, however, further advances must be made before ICG becomes an integral part of the standard management of PD.

The possible role of ICG in two other neurodegenerative diseases – namely, Huntington's disease and Alzheimer's disease – has been studied in animal models. No therapeutic applications have as yet arisen from this research, but ICG has enabled valuable insights to be gained into the pathologic processes involved. ICG is a promising tool in the investigation of epilepsy as well.

Two other topics dealt with in this issue are the use of genetically modified cells for ICG and the immunologic aspects of ICG. While knowledge of the latter is a prerequisite for successful grafting, the former opens up new avenues for exploring the central nervous system and devising therapeutic procedures.

We hope to have succeeded in our endeavor to provide the reader with extensive and up-to-date information on the restoration of brain function by means of tissue transplantation, a young branch of basic and clinical research in neuroscience.

The guest editor of this volume is Dr. Olle Lindvall (Lund, Sweden), to whose enthusiasm and efficiency I wish to pay tribute.

C. Weil
Managing Editor

Contents

Neural Transplantation in Dementia
S. B. DUNNETT

Transplantation in Experimental Epilepsy
J. BENGZON and O. LINDVALL

Genetically Modified Cells for Intracerebral Transplantation
F. H. GAGE and L. J. FISHER

Immunologic Aspects of Intracerebral CNS Tissue Transplantation
H. WIDNER

Introduction

O. Lindvall

Restorative Neurology Unit, Department of Neurology, University Hospital, Lund, Sweden

The concept of restoring function in the central nervous system (CNS) by intracerebral grafting (ICG) is not new. As long ago as the sixteenth century the famous French surgeon Ambroise Paré (1510–1590) described a patient who "... had the idea his brain was rotten. He went to the King, begging him to command M. Le Grand, Physician, M. Pigray, King's Surgeon-in-Ordinary and myself to open his head, remove his diseased brain and replace it with another. We did many things to him but it was impossible for us to restore his brain." Obviously, they did not transplant any brain tissue, or did not do so successfully, but the idea was already there over 400 years ago [3].

The era of ICG in mammals dates back to the late nineteenth century. In 1890 the New York Medical Journal contained an article by W. Gilman Thompson titled "Successful brain grafting" [7]. Large pieces of neocortical tissue had been exchanged between adult cats and dogs, and some of the grafts submitted to microscopic examination after up to 7 weeks. Despite the paper's title, the grafts probably consisted of only neuron-free remnants and scar tissue. Thompson, however, remained optimistic and concluded "I think the main fact of this experiment ... suggests an interesting field for further research, and I have no doubt that other experimenters will be rewarded in investigating it."

Almost 90 years elapsed before experimental data obtained in animals clearly suggested the possible clinical usefulness of neural grafts. It was shown in 1979 [2, 6] that the ICG of fetal dopaminergic neurons was able to reduce the signs of experimental Parkinsonism in rats. This was the first example of a functional deficit of the adult mammalian brain reversed by ICG of neurons in an animal model of a human disorder. Since then, experimental data from rodents and nonhuman primates have pointed to the potential usefulness of ICG as a new therapeutic strategy also in disorders such as Huntington's disease and dementia [5].

However, three major issues, in particular, must be taken into account when considering the potential applications in man of these animal experiments. First, how relevant is the animal model for the clinical disorder? If the pattern and distribution of pathologic changes are different in the diseased human brain, functional recovery might fail to occur after ICG. Second, how should the ICG procedure be scaled up to humans with respect both to the number of cells and implantation sites and to the location of these sites?

Third, how is graft survival and function to be assessed in patients?

How grafts may exert their functional effects is of critical importance. Four main mechanisms of action have been proposed [1]. (1) *Trophic action* (Fig. 1 c): the graft stimulates recovery mechanisms such as sprouting from intrinsic neurons. In addition to genetically engineered cells made to produce trophic factors, several types of tissue (fetal CNS, adrenal medulla, peripheral nerve) might exert a trophic effect on the host brain. (2) *Biologic minipump* (Fig. 1 d): the graft releases transmitters into the surrounding parenchyma as would a paracrine gland. This is the simplest way of correcting a biochemical deficit due to the loss of afferent, e. g., dopaminergic, neurons; its advantage over drug treatment is its action in a restricted area deprived of its intrinsic innervation. However, functional improvements might in many instances require the transmitter supply to be regulated more finely, as it is by synaptic release. Furthermore, grafts acting as biologic minipumps will probably have to be dispersed over a wide area, since the concentration of the transmitter released from a single source decreases sharply as the distance from the graft increases. (3) *Synaptic release* (Fig. 1 e): grafted neurons reinnervate the brain and form efferent synaptic contacts with the host's neurons. (4) *Integration into the host brain* (Fig. 1 f): the grafted neurons establish extensive afferent and efferent synaptic contact with the host's neurons. Several ICG models suggest that neural circuits need not be reconstructed with high precision for functional recovery to occur. Obviously, anatomic and functional integration is less likely to occur after ectopic than homotopic ICG. Dopaminergic neurons from the substantia nigra implanted into the striatum of patients with Parkinson's disease will not receive their normal afferent input; to what extent this affects the degree of functional recovery is unclear. In the excitotoxically lesioned striatum, a model for Huntington's disease, the motor and cognitive effects of grafts may depend on there being some minimal reconstruction of the "normal" neuronal circuitries.

The introduction of ICG as a possible treatment for Parkinson's disease has been prompted by the lack of an adequate medical therapy for this severe disorder. However, the ICGs performed so far in patients should not be viewed as clinical trials of procedures optimized in animals. The aim was to test whether the basic principles of cell replacement

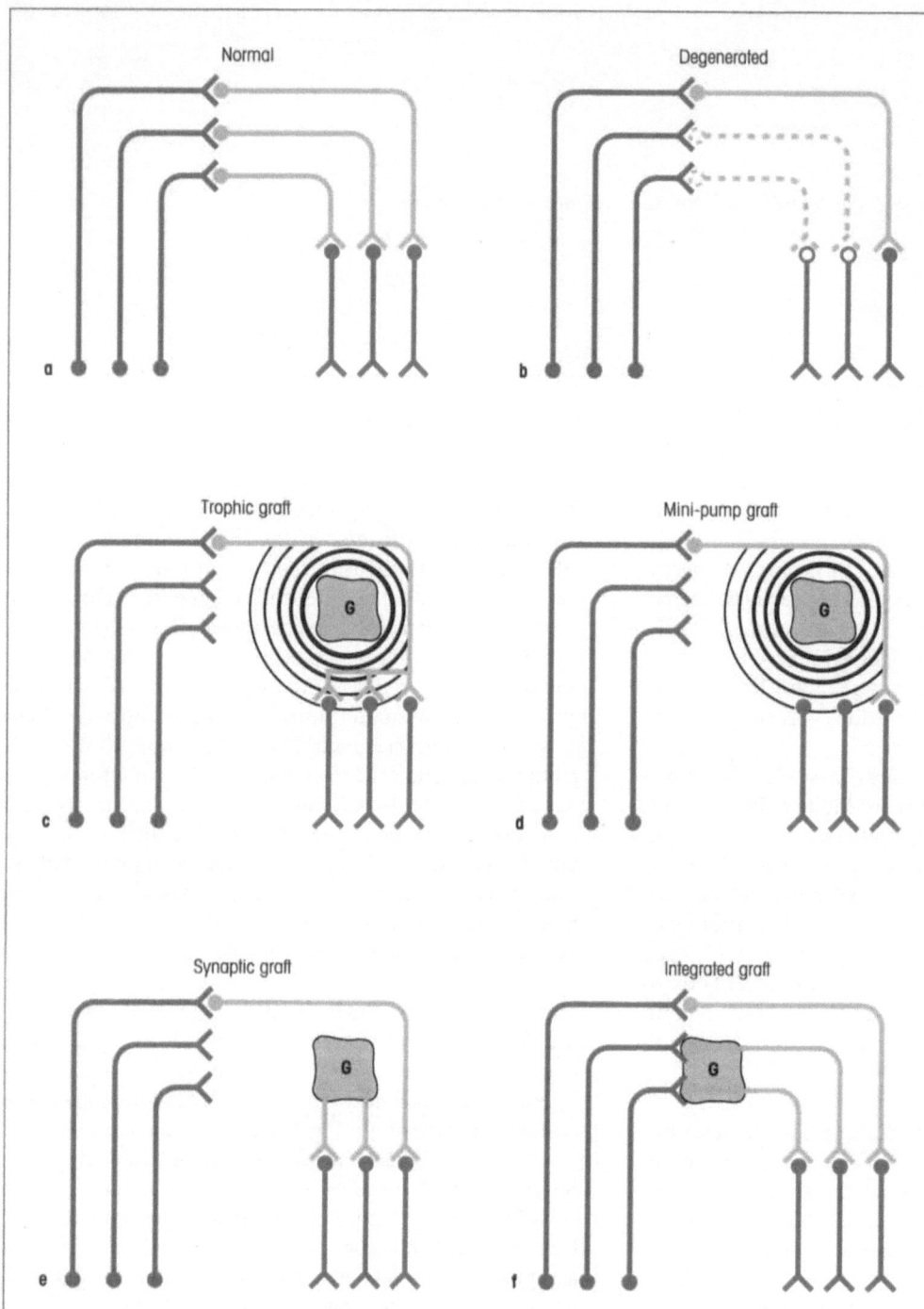

Fig. 1 a–f. *Proposed mechanism of graft-induced functional recovery after implantation into a diseased brain in which degeneration of a specific neuronal system and loss of afferent input to target neurons have occurred.*
a Normal brain, with intact neurons.
b Brain in which the degeneration of neurons deprives distal neurons of an afferent input.
c The graft stimulates recovery mechanisms in the host brain, e. g., sprouting from intrinsic neurons. All distal neurons in the figure again receive afferent input, but from a single neuron.
d The graft establishes no or very few synaptic contacts with host neurons but releases transmitters into the surrounding parenchyma, as would a paracrine gland.
e Grafted neurons reinnervate the host brain, providing distal neurons with afferent synaptic contacts and a tonic unregulated (or autoregulated) supply of transmitter sufficient to restore activation, inhibition, or disinhibition of host circuitry.
f The grafted neurons establish extensive afferent and efferent connections with the host neurons

established in animal models are valid also in the diseased human brain. The available data suggest that they are, but clearly the optimal ICG procedure for patients with Parkinson's disease has yet to be developed. The symptomatic relief observed is not such as would justify performing the procedure in a large number of patients. However, the available animal data and positive findings in patients with implants of fetal dopaminergic neurons warrant an optimistic attitude.

The source of donor tissue is a question of major importance, and human fetal neurons currently represent the best option. However, for ICG to become applicable to many patients, other cell sources will have to be found. The use of material from aborted fetuses is and will remain a controversial ethical issue, and in some countries it will not be possible (for discussion, see for instance [4] and[8]). The ICG of cells engineered genetically or enclosed in polymer capsules, secreting transmitters or neurotrophic substances, might become a clinically valuable therapeutic strategy. Until then, any attempts to use human fetal tissue must have a solid scientific basis and be performed carefully under strict ethical regulations.

The aim of this volume is to provide an overview of current research on ICG in some animal models of human neurologic disorders and to summarize the present status of ICG in humans. It will be obvious that ICG has a long way to go before it becomes a useful routine approach to treatment. The important scientific issues identified to date must be studied further in animals, but clinical studies in a few well-monitored patients will be necessary as well, since disorders such as Parkinson's or Huntington's disease do not occur in animals.

References

1. Björklund A, Lindvall O, Isacson O, Brundin P, Wictorin K, Strecker RE, Clarke DJ, Dunnett SB (1987) Mechanisms of action of intracerebral neural implants: studies on nigral and striatal grafts to the lesioned striatum. TINS 10: 509–516
2. Björklund A, Stenevi U (1979) Reconstruction of the nigrostriatal pathway by intracerebral nigral transplants. Brain Res 177: 555–560
3. Finger S (1990) A 16th century request for brain tissue transplantation. Restor Neurol Neurosci 1: 367–368
4. Hoffer BJ, Olson L (1991) Ethical issues in brain-cell transplantation. TINS 14: 384–388.
5. Lindvall O (1991) Prospects of transplantation in human neurodegenerative diseases. TINS 14: 376–384.
6. Perlow MJ, Freed WJ, Hoffer BJ, Seiger Å, Olson L, Wyatt RJ (1979) Brain grafts reduce motor abnormalities produced by destruction of nigrostriatal dopamine system. Science 204: 643–647
7. Thompson WG (1890) Successful brain grafting. NY Med J 51: 701–702
8. US Congress, Office of Technology Assessment (1990) Neural grafting: repairing the brain and spinal cord. US Government Printing Office

Transplantation in Parkinson's Disease

P. Brundin and O. Lindvall

Restorative Neurology Unit, Department of Neurology, University Hospital, Lund, Sweden

Introduction

The pathophysiologic process characteristic of Parkinson's disease (PD) is a progressive degeneration of mesostriatal dopamine (DA) neurons that eventually causes motor symptoms, primarily tremor, rigidity, and hypokinesia. Despite the marked symptomatic relief initially provided by L-dopa treatment, there is in most patients with advanced PD a progressive loss of efficacy of the drug, associated with diurnal oscillations in motor performance ("on-off" phenomena) and dyskinesias. Even though patients often temporarily benefit from changes in medication, most of them become severely incapacitated. For this large group of patients new therapeutic approaches are needed.

The clinical application of intracerebral grafting (ICG) of cells in patients with PD was first suggested in 1979, when intrastriatal implants of DA-rich ventral mesencephalic tissue from rat embryos were shown to reduce the manifestations of experimental parkinsonism in adult rats [4, 40]. Since then, studies on the DA system have played a leading role in the development of research on ICG. In addition to the obvious clinical relevance of such studies, this is probably related to several factors. First, the normal anatomy of the DA system has been mapped in detail. Second, highly sensitive and specific techniques for microscopic studies of DA neurons and their axons are available, e. g., histochemical and immunohistochemical methods for visualizing DA itself or its synthesizing enzyme tyrosine hydroxylase. Third, highly sensitive biochemical techniques are available for measuring small quantities of DA and its metabolites. Fourth, the DA system can readily be manipulated pharmacologically with drugs that release DA, inhibit its reuptake or synthesis, or stimulate or block its receptors. And fifth, specific catecholamine neurotoxins have been discovered, namely 6-hydroxydopamine (6-OHDA) and 1-methyl-4-phenyl-1,2,5,6-tetrahydropyridine (MPTP), which make it possible to deplete endogenous DA in the brain. The use of these toxins and the knowledge of DA pharmacology have led to the development of animal models of PD that are robust, sensitive, and highly suitable for assessing graft morphology and function.

Over ten years have passed since the first clinical ICG trials were performed in patients with PD, and it seems pertinent to address the question whether cell transplantation in the basal ganglia can now be regarded as an established treatment of PD and be made available to a larger number of patients. The aims of the present chapter are to answer this question, to discuss ongoing trials in the light of experimental findings in animals, and finally to describe current basic and clinical research strategies in order to proceed towards an ICG therapy in PD. Only selected references will be provided; for comprehensive reviews on ICG studies in rodents and nonhuman primates, the reader is referred to the excellent articles by Dunnett [15], Freed et al. [20], and Dunnett and Annett [16].

Experimental Studies in Animal Models of Parkinson's Disease

6-OHDA and MPTP Lesion Models

Injecting 6-OHDA into the ascending mesostriatal dopaminergic pathway can lead to an extensive degeneration of neurons in the mesencephalon and an associated loss of nerve terminals in the striatum, with a reduction of DA levels by over 95 %. Bilateral 6-OHDA lesions in rats induce a debilitating syndrome with akinesia, adipsia, and aphagia and long-lasting impairment of the initiation of spontaneous and goal-directed movements. In animals given unilateral injections, despite the intact hemisphere's maintaining normal regulatory functions there are profound motor and sensorimotor impairments on one side of the body (Fig. 1). Such animals display a spontaneous postural bias to the damaged side, towards which they turn in circles. This circling behavior can be amplified by administration of the DA-releasing agent amphetamine; the effect of DA release from the intact mesostriatal system is not opposed by DA release on the damaged side, on which there are virtually no remaining DA neurons. Administration of the directly acting DA receptor agonist apomorphine causes rotational behavior in the opposite direction, away from the lesioned side, by stimulating supersensitive DA receptors in the denervated striatum. These deficits can easily be quantified by counting the number of turns the rat performs.

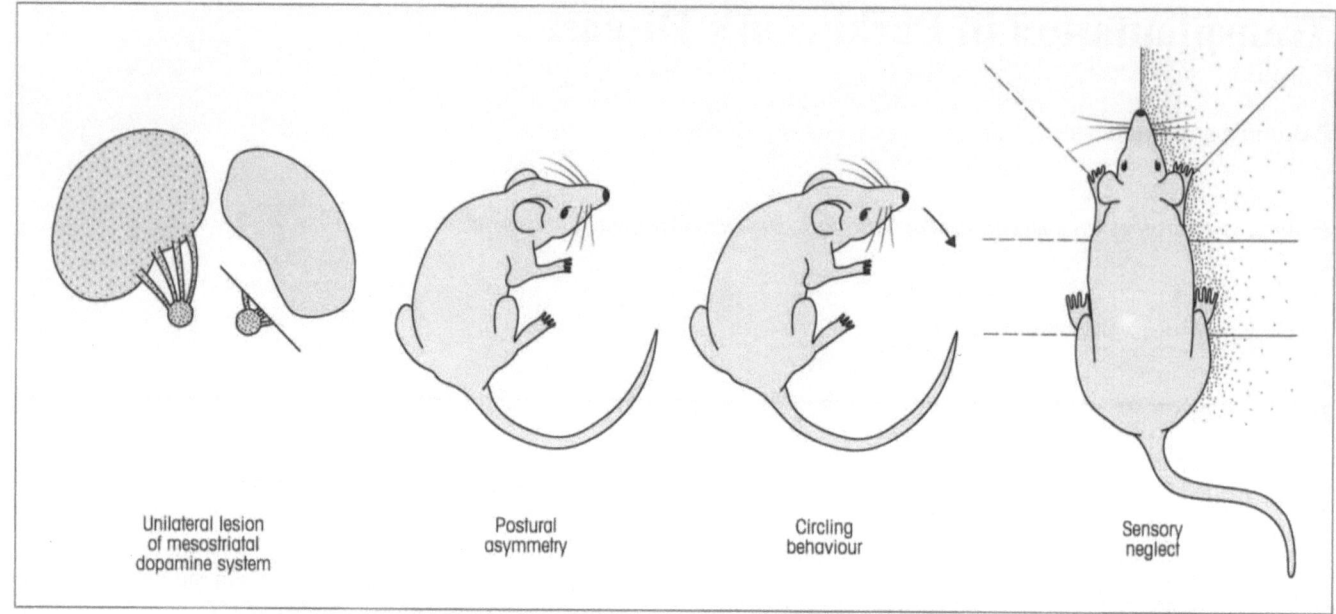

Fig. 1. *After unilateral 6-OHDA-induced lesion of the mesostriatal DA system, a quantifiable condition of hemiparkinsonism develops in the rat. It includes postural asymmetry towards the lesioned side, rotational behavior (towards the lesioned side either spontaneously or after am-* *phetamine administration, towards the nonlesioned side after apomorphine administration), and a reduced ability to respond to sensory stimuli applied to the nonlesioned side (sensory neglect)*

Rats with unilateral 6-OHDA lesions also exhibit disruption of motor responses to sensory stimuli on the side opposite the lesion ("sensory neglect," Fig. 1) and impairment of the speed, precision, and coordination of limb use on this side. Small primates, e.g., marmosets, with unilateral 6-OHDA lesions exhibit a behavioral syndrome that includes several of the features observed in rats.

The rat with a unilateral lesion of the DA system provides a most useful model in which to study the morphologic development and functional capacity of grafted DA neurons. Even though rats with bilateral lesions seem to present a closer analogy to clinical parkinsonism, they have the disadvantage of suffering from aphagia and adipsia, which make tube feeding necessary.

In 1982 a group of young heroin addicts injected themselves with a synthetic pethidine derivative contaminated with MPTP, and within a few days severe and persistent signs of parkinsonism developed. MPTP has since been used in experimental research as a tool to generate animal models of PD. The toxin is particularly effective in primates, less so in rodents. MPTP is administered to primates either systemically to induce bilateral lesions or into a carotid artery or the CNS to induce unilateral lesions. It causes selective destruction of the dopaminergic neurons in the substantia nigra, pars compacta, and a consequent severe DA depletion in the striatum. This leads to the development of cardinal signs of human PD such as rigidity, tremor, and hypokinesia. One problem with this model is the large interindividual variability in the response to the drug and the unpredictable spontaneous recovery of behavioral deficits and biochemical markers that occurs in some ani-

mals. Notwithstanding these shortcomings, the MPTP-treated nonhuman primate has proved to be useful for studies on the functional capacity of grafted cells in higher species.

Grafting of Embryonic Dopamine Neurons

Various methods have been used to implant embryonic DA-rich mesencephalic tissue into the rat brain. Solid pieces have been placed in the lateral ventricle or, alternatively, into a cavity prepared in the neocortex adjacent to the striatum. In most studies, the donor tissue has been dissociated prior to grafting and implanted, in the form of a cell suspension, into one or several striatal sites by stereotaxic injection (Fig. 2). The donor tissue has to be embryonic/fetal in order for the grafted DA neurons to survive; older tissue is probably too susceptible to mechanical trauma and anoxia to survive. The upper age limit for rat donor tissue is about 17 days after conception with the solid-graft technique and 15–16 days after conception with the cell-suspension method. When human DA neurons are grafted into rats with experimental parkinsonism, a similar difference in upper age limit seems to apply: 12 weeks after conception for solid grafts and 8 weeks after conception for dissociated grafts.

Despite their surviving well in most sites in the rat brain, grafted DA neurons extend numerous axons only when implanted close to or directly into their normal target area (Fig. 3). In the denervated rat striatum, mesencephalic grafts can give rise to a dopaminergic innervation having

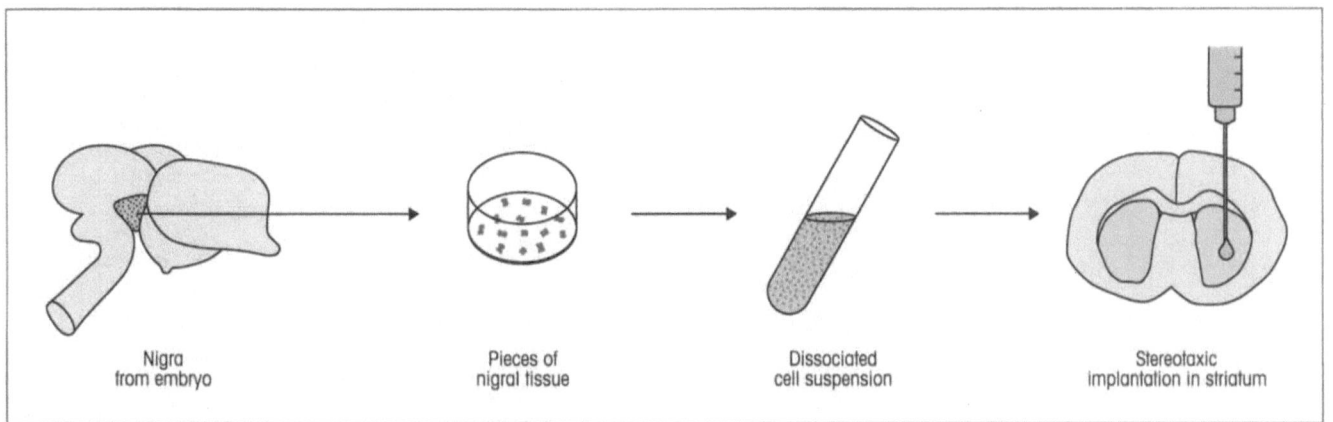

Fig. 2. *The routine transplantation technique for dissociated embryonic neurons involves several steps. First, the ventral mesencephalon is dissected from embryos. Second, tissue from several embryos is pooled and incubated with trypsin at 37 °C for 20 min. Third, following rinsing the tissue is mechanically dissociated with a Pasteur pipette. Finally, portions of the dissociated mesencephalic tissue are injected stereotaxically into the desired region(s) by means of a microsyringe*

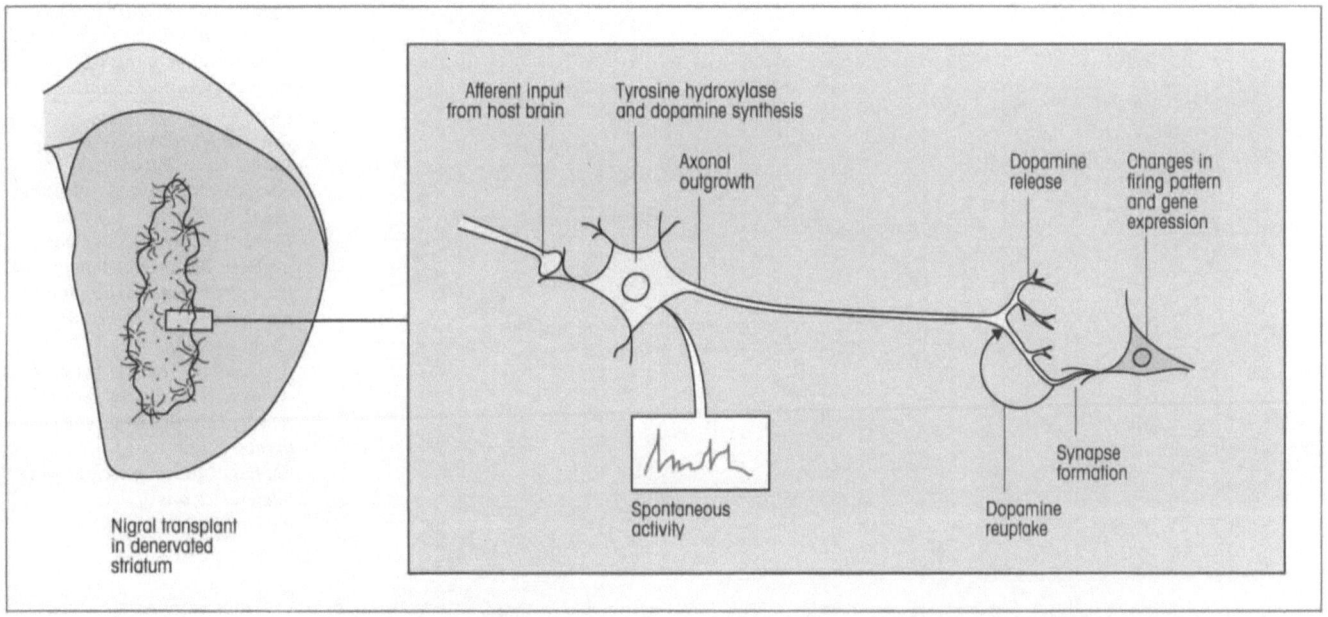

Fig. 3. *Grafted embryonic DA neurons display several of the morphologic and physiologic features of normal DA neurons: they form synaptic contacts with host striatal neurons, receive afferents from the host, release DA spontaneously, and display electric activity*

about 50% of its normal density in the immediate vicinity of the graft and tapering off to about 20% at a distance of 1.0 mm from the graft [13]. Electron microscopic studies have shown that the DA fibers also form synapses with host striatal cells and that dendrites from grafted cells make synaptic contact with axons of presumed host origin. Serotoninergic fibers originating in the host raphe and corticostriatal fibers coming from the host frontal cortex innervate parts of the mesencephalic grafts. However, the innervation from the host striatum, a region that normally heavily innervates the substantia nigra, is sparse. Electric stimulation of the cortex, raphe, and striatum of the host leads to changes in the activity of cells in mesencephalic grafts. Even in their ectopic location in the striatum instead of the substantia

nigra, the grafted DA neurons may thus receive a regulatory input from the host brain.

Mesencephalic grafts can restore the DA levels in a completely denervated rat striatum to a mean of 6%–18% of normal levels. Furthermore, there is a 50%–100% increase in DOPAC to DA ratio (DOPAC, i.e., dihydroxyphenylacetic acid, is a major metabolite of DA), indicating a higher DA turnover in the grafts than in the normal mesostriatal DA system. In vivo microdialysis studies have shown that DA is released spontaneously (Fig. 3), and at a higher rate than normal, from graft-derived terminals. Spontaneously active DA neurons have been detected in intraventricular grafts of mesencephalic tissue also by means of electrophysiologic methods (Fig. 3). As do normal neurons, the grafts

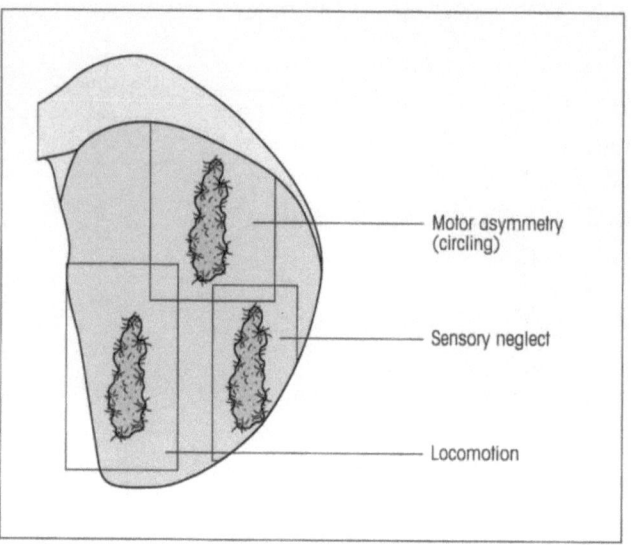

Fig. 4. *Grafts of embryonic DA neurons affect the 6-OHDA-induced hemiparkinsonian syndrome in the rat in different ways according to which part of the host striatum their fibers reinnervate. Grafts placed in the dorsal caudate-putamen reverse motor asymmetry (rotation); grafts innervating the ventrolateral caudate-putamen reduce sensory neglect; and implants located in the nucleus accumbens increase locomotion*

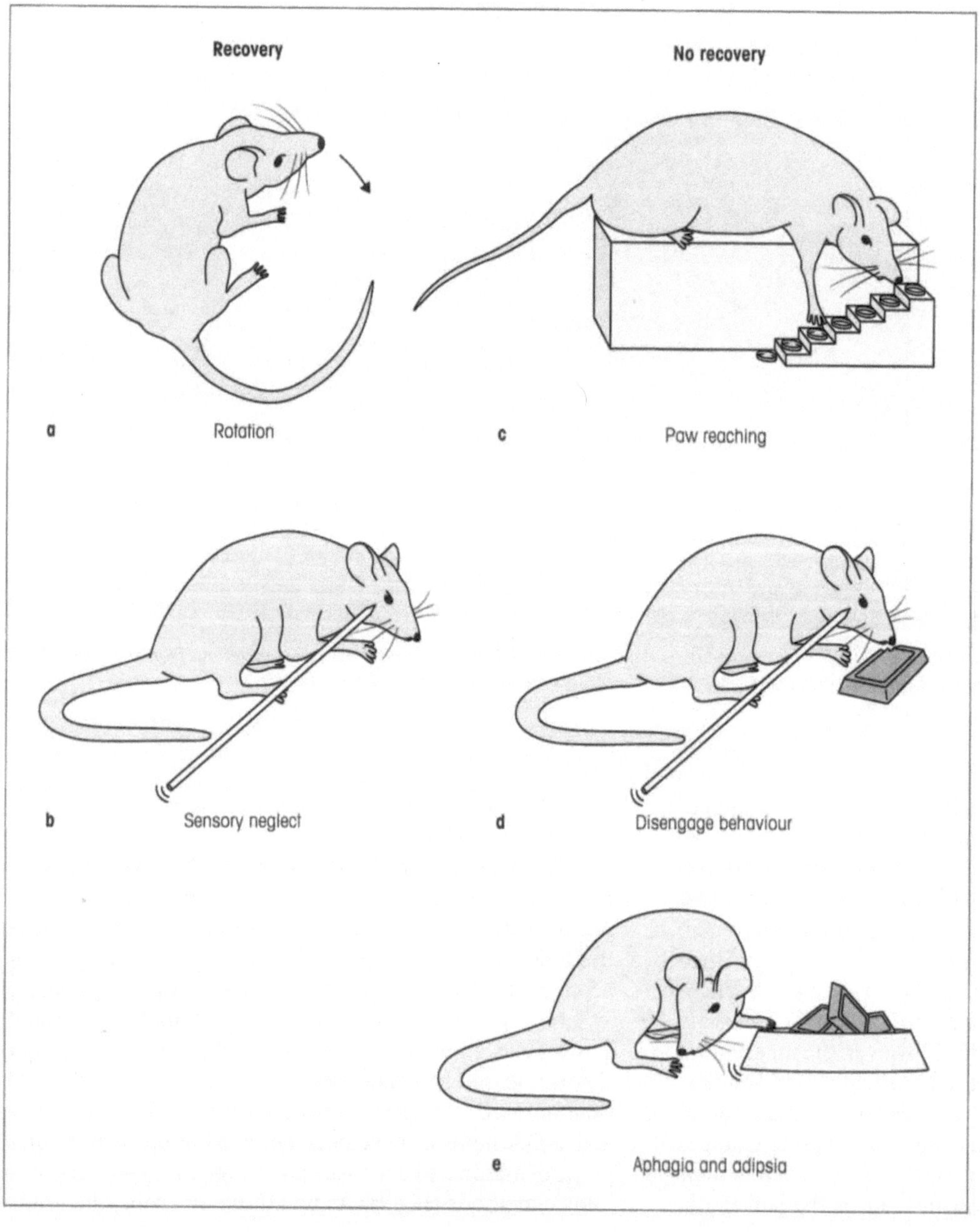

Motor asymmetry (circling)

Sensory neglect

Locomotion

Recovery

No recovery

a   Rotation

c   Paw reaching

b   Sensory neglect

d   Disengage behaviour

e   Aphagia and adipsia

Fig. 5 a–e. *Behavioral deficits significantly reversed by DA-rich mesencephalic grafts placed in the striatum of rats with experimental parkinsonism include*
a motor asymmetry, both spontaneous and after administration of DA-releasing agents (amphetamine), and
b sensorimotor deficits (sensory neglect). Behavioral deficits that it has so far not been possible to ameliorate significantly include
c paw reaching;
d "disengage" behavior, i. e., the ability to respond to a perioral sensory stimulus while engaged in eating; and
e aphagia and adipsia following bilateral lesions of the mesostriatal DA system

respond to amphetamine administration with a severalfold increase of DA release, their DA reuptake system is blocked by nomifensine, and they exhibit autoregulatory features since their DA release is decreased by the receptor agonist apomorphine. In the host striatum, the graft-derived innervation causes postsynaptic DA-binding sites to return to normal density.

Grafts of embryonic DA neurons are able to reverse both spontaneous and drug-induced rotational behavior in rats with a unilateral 6-OHDA lesion of the mesostriatal system (Fig. 4 and 5) [4, 40]. These effects are dependent on the DA-neuron component in the transplants and disappear if the grafts are destroyed. Interestingly, only a few percent of the normal number of DA cells and of the normal striatal DA level need to be restored by the grafts for compensation of amphetamine-evoked rotational asymmetry. The underlying reason(s) could be one or several of the following: (1) the host neurons in the denervated striatum have become supersensitive to DA; (2) the grafted DA neurons exhibit increased DA turnover and release; (3) amphetamine administration increases the efficacy of the system by creating an abnormal situation with greatly increased transmitter release; (4) the area critical for rotational behavior seems to be restricted to a minor part of the dorsolateral striatum (Fig. 4), i. e., the target insertion site for the graft. The clinical implications of these findings are that functional improvements in patients might be induced by grafts that restore only a small fraction of the normal striatal DA innervation.

The effects of ICG on different components of the 6-OHDA-induced hemiparkinsonian syndrome in rats seem to depend upon the striatal region being reinnervated by the grafts (Fig. 4). Thus, grafts innervating the dorsal striatum reverse rotational asymmetry but do not affect deficits in sensorimotor orientation. Conversely, grafts reinnervating the ventrolateral striatum reverse the latter impairment but leave rotational asymmetry unchanged. When DA neurons are implanted into the denervated nucleus accumbens, they can restore normal amphetamine-induced locomotor activity.

Considerably fewer anatomic and functional data are available from ICG studies in monkeys. Several reports have provided evidence for the survival of dopaminergic neurons, the reinnervation of the host striatum, and the functional effects of grafts of embryonic mesencephalic tissue placed in either the caudate or putamen of MPTP- or 6-OHDA-lesioned primates (for references, see [16]). Both solid implants and cell suspensions have been used. In animals with surviving grafts there has been a reduction in parkinsonian symptoms including rigidity, tremor, and hypokinesia. However, whereas these studies have confirmed in primates the basic findings made in rodents of the survival and functional capacity of neural grafts, they have provided little new information on issues of major clinical relevance. Such issues include, for instance, immunologic aspects, problems of scaling up the procedure to innervate the larger primate striatum, the question whether only some or most of the symptoms of PD can be improved, and the relative functional importance of different implantation sites (cau-

date, putamen, and/or other structures). Only in recent studies on marmosets with unilateral 6-OHDA lesions of the mesostriatal pathway have grafts in the caudate nucleus and in the putamen – two structures that are anatomically distinct in primates – been systematically compared with each other. Dunnett and Annett [16] found that grafts in the caudate nucleus reversed drug-induced rotation whereas grafts in the putamen improved contralateral limb use, neither graft alone being able to affect both types of deficit.

Many symptoms in animals with experimental parkinsonism can be alleviated or even abolished by grafts of embryonic DA neurons, but others cannot, even in rats (Fig. 5). Whereas DA-rich grafts cause recovery of 6-OHDA-lesioned rats in simple sensory or motor behavioral tests and tests of drug-induced behavior, they induce no improvement in many complex motor and sensorimotor tasks. In a test called "disengage behavior," the rats are poked with a probe in the perioral region while eating chocolate; a normal rat responds by turning its head towards the sensory stimulus and biting the probe, while rats with unilateral 6-OHDA lesions continue to eat for a prolonged time and seem to be unable to switch their attention ("disengage") to the new stimulus. Interestingly, a rat with a graft of DA neurons in the ventrolateral striatum displays recovery in the simple sensorimotor orientation test in which it is required to orient toward the sensory stimulus while not engaged in another activity, but does not exhibit any improvement in the disengage test [35]. Besides, grafts do not reverse the deficit in the use of the contralateral forelimbs for discrete skilled movements that is caused by unilateral lesions of the mesostriatal DA system [18] or the aphagia and adipsia caused by bilateral 6-OHDA lesions [17]. It has been speculated that the inability of a graft to reverse a particular functional deficit is due to a limited integration of the grafted cells in the host brain; this hypothesis is supported by findings that grafts in neonatal rats, in which neuronal plasticity is believed to be greater, can prevent aphagia and adipsia [45]. The differential sensitivity of symptoms to graft-induced recovery in 6-OHDA-lesioned rats could have important clinical correlates: thus, mesencephalic grafts may alleviate some, but not all, symptoms of PD in humans.

In recent years there has been a great deal of discussion over the mechanisms of functional recovery. The debate has focused on whether the functional changes observed after ICG are due to reinnervation from DA neurons in the grafts or to the sprouting of axons from the host DA system. In animals with 6-OHDA-induced parkinsonism there is nearly no residual DA innervation in the striatum (usually less than 1 % of normal), which leaves virtually no host DA system as a substratum for a putative sprouting mechanism. In such animals, the survival of the grafted DA neurons, their fiber outgrowth, and their releasing DA in the brain are likely to be of critical importance for the functional effects. The situation may be different in MPTP-treated animals, in which part of the striatal DA innervation is usually spared, particularly that originating in the medially located DA neurons in the ventral tegmental area [3]. As proposed, for instance, by Bankiewicz et al. [3], this spared input may respond to the

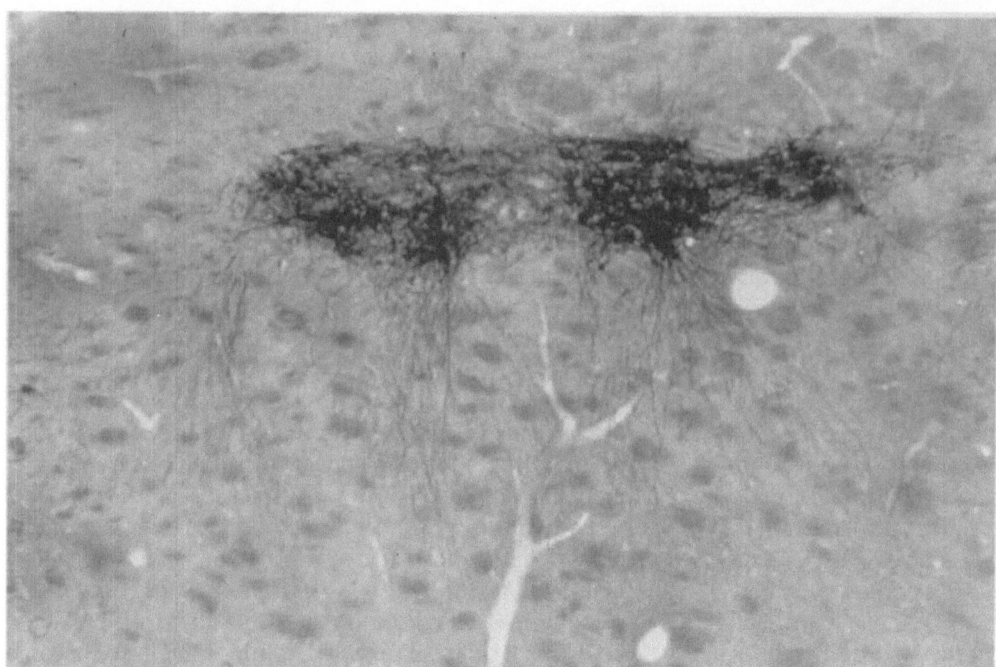

Fig. 6. *Photomicrograph showing a human embryonic mesencephalic transplant rich in DA neurons stained with an antibody against the DA-synthesizing enzyme tyrosine hydroxylase. The grafted neurons extended numerous fibers into the previously denervated rat striatum. In this particular rat, the motor symptoms caused by a 6-OHDA-induced lesion of the mesostriatal DA system were reversed by the graft*

ICG by sprouting or increased DA synthesis and thus contribute to the recovery of DA transmission in the host striatum; the ICG surgery itself (i.e., the act of creating a cavity in the caudate nucleus) can induce moderate sprouting, which is further enhanced by surviving grafts consisting of both neuronal and nonneuronal tissues. Some of the functional effects achieved may, accordingly, be due in part to neurotrophic activities induced by surgery and in part to factors secreted by the graft that promote neurite outgrowth. However, even if sprouting-induced recovery remains an interesting possibility, it remains to be demonstrated consistently and its functional significance to be clarified; at any rate, it is unlikely to be operative in animals or humans having sustained a nearly complete loss of the striatal DA innervation.

Human Embryonic Dopamine Neurons Grafted into the Rat Brain

In order to assess several parameters of critical importance for the clinical application of DA neuron grafting, human embryonic brain tissue – ventral mesencephalic tissue from donors aged 6.5–19 weeks – has been implanted into immunosuppressed 6-OHDA-lesioned rats [7, 9]. The human DA neurons, prepared as cell suspensions, survived xenografting well only when taken from embryos aged 8 weeks after conception or younger. Even then, the survival rate of the implanted DA neurons was probably in the same low range as for rat donor tissue (about 5%). When the grafts were implanted as solid pieces, surviving DA neurons were observed also in tissue obtained from 12-week-

old fetuses [46, 47]. The grafted DA neurons gave rise to an extensive terminal network in the whole of the rat striatum (Fig. 6) and formed synapses with host striatal neurons [9, 10, 46]. At 12–20 weeks after ICG surgery, the human mesencephalic grafts reversed both spontaneous and drug-induced motor asymmetry in the recipient hemiparkinsonian rats [7, 9, 24, 47] and also displayed spontaneous DA release [9]. Electrophysiologic recordings revealed spontaneously active dopaminergic neurons within the graft and host striatal firing rates consistent with those of DA-innervated cells [24, 49].

In summary, (1) human embryonic DA neurons survive ICG to the rat, reinnervate the host striatum, are spontaneously active and release DA, and can reverse symptoms of experimental parkinsonism; (2) optimal donor age is 6–8 weeks after conception when the ventral mesencephalon is prepared according to the dissociated-tissue technique.

Grafting of Adrenal Medulla

The strategy of implanting catecholamine-rich, chromaffin adrenal medullary (AM) tissue into the DA-denervated striatum avoids both the ethical issues involved in the use of human embryonic tissue and the problems of immunologic rejection, since the graft tissue can be taken from one of the patient's own adrenal glands (autograft).

Most studies of this type have been conducted in unilaterally 6-OHDA-lesioned rats. In general, AM cells survive poorly after direct implantation into the striatal parenchyma. The survival is better, although still variable, when the tissue is placed in the adjacent lateral ventricle. Normal chromaffin cells secrete primarily epinephrine and only low amounts of DA. However, in long-term intraventricular AM grafts, DA and norepinephrine are the predominant catecholamines, a fact suggesting that transplantation causes a shift in secretory activity. There is almost no fiber outgrowth from the implanted chromaffin cells, probably because of an inadequate activity of nerve growth factor (NGF) in the adult striatum. Adding NGF to the graft, preferably by continuous intrastriatal infusion over several weeks, significantly increases cell survival, causes a transformation of many cells towards a more neuronal phenotype, and greatly enhances the fiber outgrowth into the host striatum [48]. There appears to be a need for a constant NGF supply to maintain this graft-derived fiber plexus [48].

The survival of chromaffin tissue after grafting has been poor also in MPTP-treated nonhuman primates. Two procedures recently described possibly increase its survival: stereotaxic intrastriatal implantation of long, narrow ribbons of tissue [14] and cografting with a segment of peripheral (e. g., sural) nerve, which is believed to act as a biologic source of NGF [27].

The functional effects of AM transplantation in rats and monkeys seem to alleviate only drug-induced rotational asymmetry, without affecting spontaneous behavior. AM grafts have far less effect on rotational behavior than DA-rich mesencephalic tissue [6], and their functional effects are transient over a few weeks if no NGF is supplied. The infusion of NGF will increase their duration of action [48], but the grafts tend to die and the functional effects disappear after the NGF infusion is stopped. A few studies on the functional capacity of AM grafts in MPTP-treated monkeys have been reported. Plunkett et al. [41] found a reduction of apomorphine-induced rotational asymmetry after AM transplantation into a cavity prepared in the caudate nucleus, but the same effect was observed with cavitation alone. The improvement was not as complete as after fetal dopaminergic grafts.

There is little evidence to support the hypothesis that the functional effects after AM transplantation in animals are due to catecholamine release from the grafts. No spontaneous catecholamine release could be detected from intrastriatal implants of chromaffin cells by in vivo electrochemistry [12], and reductions in apomorphine-induced rotation similar to those observed with AM grafts were achieved with grafts of tissues not producing catecholamines, e. g., adipose tissue or sciatic nerve, supplemented with NGF infusions [42].

As in the case of embryonic DA neurons (see above), it has been suggested that the functional capacity of AM grafts is related to their inducing trophic responses in the host brain. When chromaffin cells are injected into the striatum of MPTP-treated mice or monkeys with a partial lesion of the DA system, there is an increased immunostaining for the DA-synthesizing enzyme tyrosine hydroxylase [5]. The underlying mechanism and the functional consequences are unclear, and the phenomenon may be related to the tissue trauma.

Clinical Studies in Patients with Parkinson's Disease

Grafting of Adrenal Medulla

The first clinical trials with AM autotransplantation were carried out between 1982 and 1985 by means of stereotaxic ICG in four patients with PD. Only minor and transient improvements, lasting for a couple of months, were seen after unilateral grafting to either the caudate nucleus or the putamen [2, 28]. The major interest in this approach arose from the study by Madrazo et al. [33], in which they reported successful AM autotransplantation in two young patients with PD. Instead of a stereotaxic approach, the authors used open microsurgical techniques and implanted pieces of AM tissue through the cerebral cortex into a cavity prepared in the head of the caudate nucleus on one side. Madrazo et al. [34] have summarized their findings up to 1–3 years postoperatively in 42 consecutive patients. Four patients died, and another four could not be followed up. Assessed by means of different rating scales, the response was good in 60 % of the remaining 34 patients, moderate in 20 %, and poor in only 20 %. The improvement had a gradual onset, was always bilateral, and affected mainly rigidity, bradykinesia, postural instability, and gait disturbances. The mean dose of L-dopa could be reduced by 60 %.

Other groups, however, have not observed any dramatic improvement after AM autotransplantation (for references see [20]). From a series of 61 patients [21] comparable to those operated on by Madrazo et al. [34], 2-year follow-up data were collected on 56 patients subjected to AM autotransplantation by stereotaxic surgery or open craniotomy. Eleven patients died, and half of these deaths were possibly related to the surgery. The patients showed a significant, though modest, reduction of the severity and duration of off periods but remained very incapacitated. The doses of antiparkinsonian medication could not be reduced. Two years after surgery, only about 32 % of survivors remained improved, and 22 % had persistent psychiatric morbidity.

Most investigators agree that the further development of intracerebral AM transplantation should be pursued primarily in the laboratory. Even with the microsurgical procedure, only modest improvements have been achieved in about 30 %–50 % of patients, who still had motor fluctuations. Importantly, the morbidity and mortality have been considerable. As to the mechanisms of improvement, there is no evidence to support the notion that it could be due to the expected catecholamine release from implanted cells. In fact, few or no transplanted catecholamine-producing chromaffin cells have been found to have survived in autopsied patients [23, 26].

Grafting of Embryonic Dopamine Neurons

Over 100 patients with PD have so far received implants of human embryonic mesencephalic tissue into the striatum,

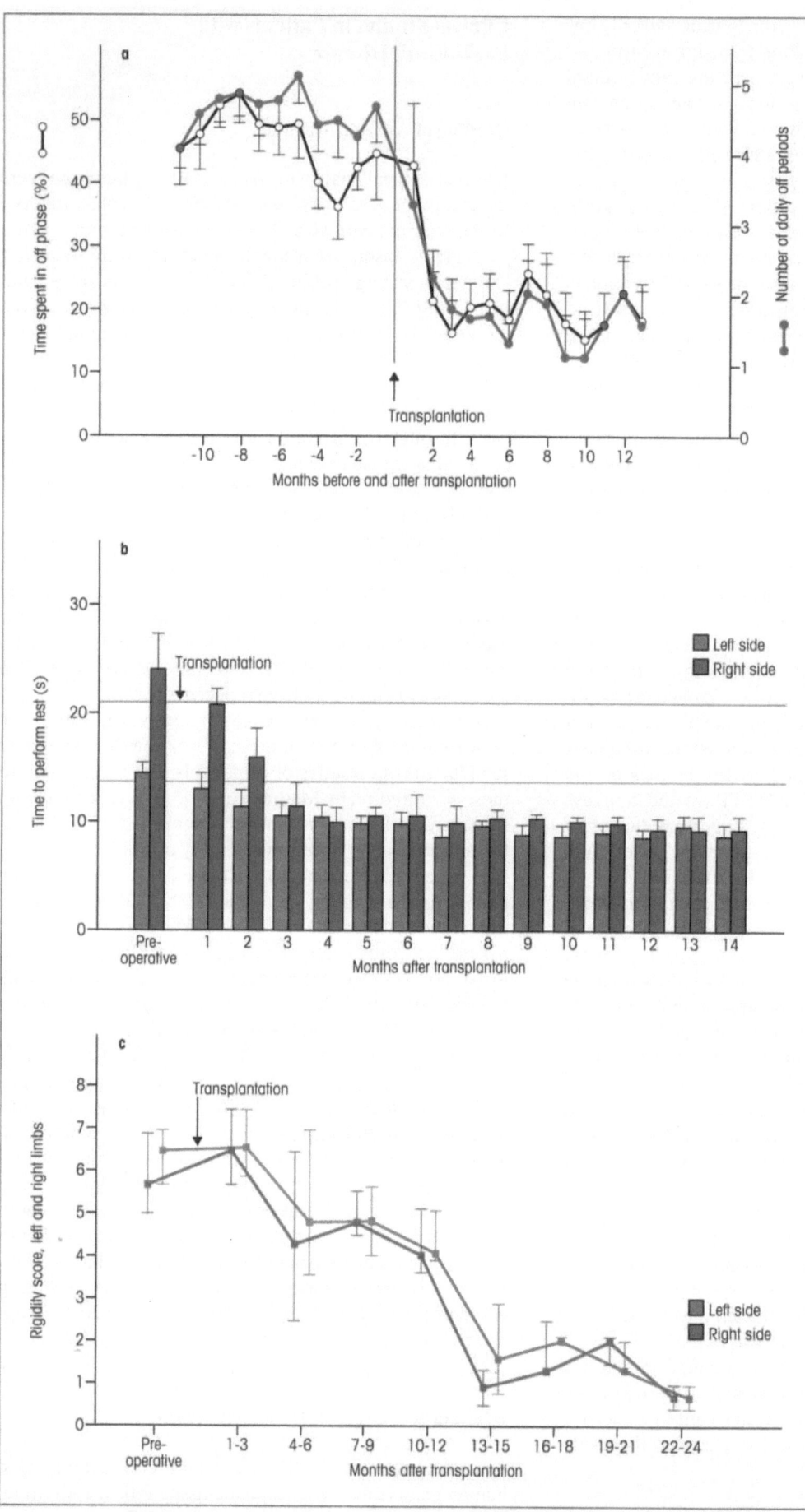

Fig. 7 a–c. Illustration that neural grafting can effect a sustained improvement of motor function in PD.

a, b Motor performance in a patient with idiopathic PD who received implants of ventral mesencephalic tissue from four aborted embryos (age 6–7 weeks after conception) at three sites in the left putamen.

a Mean monthly percentage of time spent awake per day with parkinsonian symptoms (off phases) and mean number of daily off periods for 11 months before and 14 months after transplantation (based on daily self-scoring by the patient). The bars show 99 % confidence limits. During the second and subsequent postoperative months, there was a marked reduction of both the time spent in off phases and the number of daily off periods.

b Time taken to perform 20 pronations-supinations with the left and the right arm while in the off state. From the second month after transplantation, the task was performed more rapidly than it had been preoperatively. The improvement was bilateral but more pronounced on the right side (contralateral to the graft). The vertical bars show the means of measurements and 99 % confidence limits. The horizontal lines show the preoperative means minus confidence limits for the left (blue line) and the right (red line) arm.

c Rigidity score in a patient with MPTP-induced parkinsonism who received bilateral implants at one site in the caudate and three sites in the putamen; tissue from three to four aborted embryos was grafted on each side. Sum of rigidity scores in the wrist, elbow, and knee on the left (blue curve) and the right (red curve) side, respectively. From about 1 year postoperatively, there is a marked bilateral reduction in rigidity. Median values ±25 percentiles

Fig. 8. Serial positron emission tomography (PET) scans obtained with 6-L-(^{18}F)-fluorodopa at two similar anatomic levels through the caudate and putamen of the patient whose motor performance is shown in Fig. 7 a, b. The scans show activity 12 months before and 5, 8, and 13 months after grafting. Each image has been scaled to the activity recorded in the occipital cortex, in order that sequential studies may be compared directly. A clear focal increase is seen in the left putamen, into which the grafts had been placed. Kinetic data indicate that the uptake of 6-L-(^{18}F)-fluorodopa continued to increase for up to 8 months in the putamen operated on, despite a progressive fall in tracer uptake in striatal structures not operated on

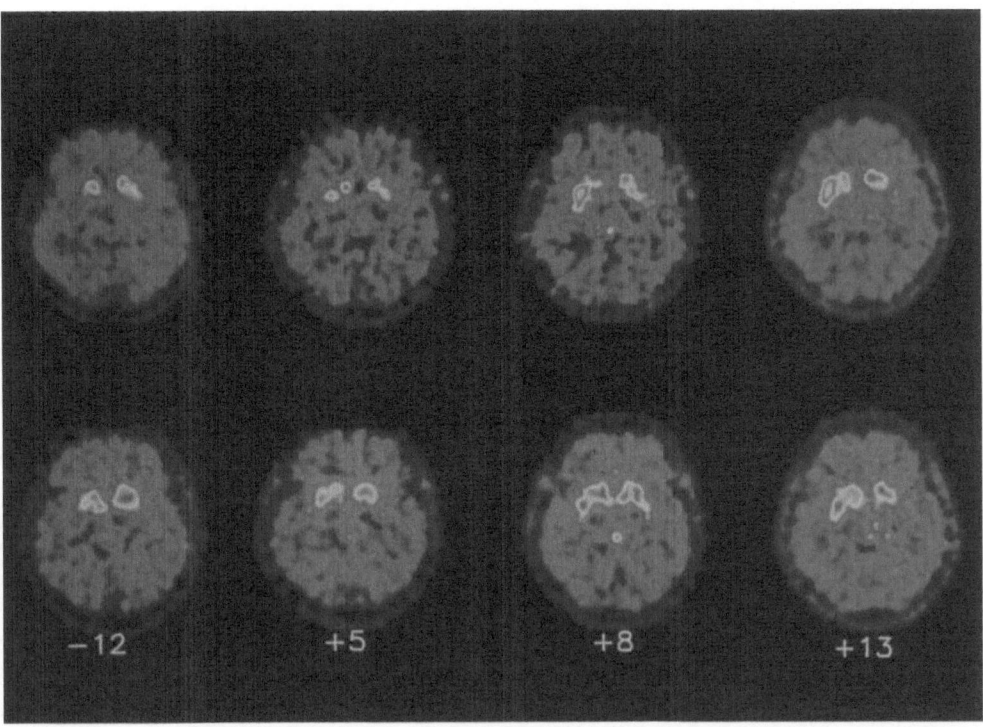

either by stereotaxic ICG of dissociated tissue directly into the striatum or by placement of pieces or fragments of nigral tissue into a cavity in the head of the caudate nucleus. The grafts have been placed unilaterally, in a few cases bilaterally, at one to ten target sites per side in the caudate nucleus and/or putamen. In most studies, tissue from a single embryo has been used in each patient, but Lindvall et al. [29–31] implanted tissue from four embryos on one side; the same amount of tissue was grafted on each side in two patients with MPTP-induced parkinsonism described by Widner et al. [51]. Embryonic ages have ranged from 6 to 19 weeks. Most patients have been subjected to immunosuppressive treatment.

The reported data [19, 22, 29–32, 34, 36, 44, 51] can be summarized as follows: (1) Minor to moderate improvement of motor symptoms has been observed in almost all patients, but in no case has there been a full reversal of symptomatology. (2) Improvements consisted of a prolonged duration of response to L-dopa, an increased percentage time spent in on phase, and a reduction of the severity of symptoms, particularly during off phases (Fig. 7). (3) Regarding individual symptoms, tremor has shown little change, whereas the most consistent improvement has been observed for rigidity and hypo-/bradykinesia. (4) The latent period before the onset of improvement has ranged from nil (onset immediately after ICG) to 3–6 months, and further improvement has occurred for up to 30 months after grafting. In the two patients with MPTP-induced parkinsonism,

further symptomatic relief was observed for up to at least 24 months [51]. (5) No significant adverse effects have been registered. (6) Finally, evidence for a survival of grafted DA neurons has been provided in only four patients. Positron emission tomography (PET) has demonstrated a significant increase of 6-L-(^{18}F)-fluorodopa uptake in the host striatum in four patients who improved clinically (Fig. 8) [30, 31, 44, 51]; since there is no evidence for a breakdown of the blood-brain barrier [31, 44], the most likely explanation is that the grafts restore DA synthesis and storage in the striatum. This is probably due to survival and growth of the grafted embryonic DA neurons, but a trophic effect of the embryonic tissue leading to axonal sprouting of the host's own DA system cannot be entirely excluded.

In conclusion, the clinical trials reported so far indicate that embryonic neural tissue can be implanted into the human brain without major risks. Improvements have ·been observed, but even in the best cases no complete reversal of multiple or single parkinsonian symptoms has been obtained. The results from the various groups are difficult to compare because of differences in design (duration of preoperative assessment period, drug regimens, methods of evaluation) and lack of data on graft survival in most patients. Variations in the design also make it difficult to draw conclusions about the relative importance for graft survival of factors such as the surgical and tissue preparation techniques, the number of implantation sites, the number and age of embryos, and the use of immunosuppression.

Research Strategies for the Development of a Transplantation Therapy in Parkinson's Disease

Adrenal Medulla

The development of AM autotransplantation into a useful treatment for patients with PD necessitates two major advances. First, the morbidity and mortality rates of the surgical procedure must be considerably reduced. Fewer complications seem to occur, for instance, with a retroperitoneal than with a transperitoneal approach for adrenalectomy and with a stereotaxic procedure than with open craniotomy for tissue implantation [21]. Second, the symptomatic relief achieved has to be markedly increased. However, little is known on how AM grafts act. Much interest has recently been focused on the hypothesis that AM tissue contains some unknown trophic factor(s) or that the ICG surgery induces the formation of such a factor, able to stimulate axonal sprouting from the DA neurons remaining in the host. Morphologic support for this phenomenon has been provided by autopsy studies in two PD patients subjected to AM grafting [23, 26]. Still, the functional importance of the presumed sprouting-derived new striatal innervation is unknown at present and must be investigated in animal experiments. Recently, the possible involvement of basic fibroblast growth factor (bFGF) has been suggested, since this factor, present in both the adrenal gland and the brain, increases in areas of injury and promotes the survival and neurite extension of DA neurons in culture. In support of this idea, Otto and Unsicker [39] have shown that bFGF can stimulate the recovery of nigral DA neurons in MPTP-treated mice.

Another strategy, namely increasing the capacity of the grafts to secrete DA and other catecholamines, requires that the long-term survival of AM cells be substantially improved. This is currently being attempted by supplying the graft tissue with NGF. As described above, animal studies have shown that NGF supplied by infusion [48], cografts of NGF-secreting peripheral nerve [27], or genetically engineered cells [11] significantly increases the number of surviving chromaffin cells. On the basis of these data, clinical programs of AM autotransplantation plus NGF supply have been initiated. One patient, who received NGF by intrastriatal infusion for 4 weeks after the stereotaxic ICG of AM cells, has been described to exhibit improved motor function, although the result was modest [38]. Other series of patients are currently receiving double grafts of AM cells and peripheral nerve, but no data are yet available.

Embryonic Dopamine Neurons

The demonstration that grafts of human embryonic DA neurons can survive and exert functional effects in the parkinsonian brain is only the first step towards an ICG therapy. Achieving a more complete functional recovery entails improving the ICG procedure, e.g., by increasing the number of transplantation sites, the survival of grafted DA neurons, their volume of reinnervation within the striatum, and possibly also their integration into the host brain. In addition, graft placement outside the caudate-putamen might be required for optimal symptomatic relief. For long-term graft survival, efficient suppression of adverse immune responses is probably necessary (see the chapter by Widner, this volume).

Only 5%–20% of human or rat DA neurons survive ICG into rats with the dissociated-tissue technique [9, 43]. The reason for the marked cell loss is not understood. It may be related to acute cell trauma during the dissection and tissue preparation, prolonged anoxia, or lack of trophic factors in the adult host brain. Attempts to increase DA neuron survival in animal experiments by supplying the grafts with trophic factors such as bFGF, brain-derived neurotrophic factor (BDNF), and NGF, with the calcium channel antagonist nimodipine or with monoganglioside GM1 have so far yielded no major increase in survival rate.

On the basis of the results from human-to-rat grafting experiments, we now estimate that the implantation of ventral mesencephalic tissue from one human embryo into the caudate nucleus or putamen of a patient with PD might be able to restore up to 15%–20% of the number of cells normally innervating either of these structures. In confirmation of this, serial PET scans showed high fluorodopa uptake at the implantation sites in two patients who had received grafts into the putamen of mesencephalic tissue from four embryos each [44]. It seems unlikely that increasing the number of surviving DA neurons at each implantation site would lead to further clinical improvement in these patients. The volume of the striatum is about 200 times greater in the human than in the rat brain, and even a large number of surviving neurons might fail to produce an adequate volume of graft-derived innervation. The extent of striatal reinnervation is dependent not only on DA neuron survival but also on the number and location of implantation sites and on the growth capacity of DA neurons. When grafted into the rat striatum, human DA neurons have exhibited a higher growth capacity than rat DA neurons, but the maximal extension of their axonal processes is not known. We have estimated that, if human embryonic DA neurons are implanted along three tracts in the putamen (as was done in four of our patients), still only about 25% of the total volume of this structure would be reached by a graft-derived reinnervation with a density 25% or more of normal. In a nearly completely denervated human parkinsonian brain, a DA terminal density of 25% could represent a critical level for obtaining functional effects. Two strategies might be envisaged to achieve more complete reinnervation of the striatal complex: first, the graft material could be distributed more efficiently over larger areas and bilaterally – but this could carry an additional surgical risk; second, the graft tissue might be supplied with a trophic factor such as bFGF or BDNF before and/or after ICG, in order to enhance the axonal outgrowth of mesencephalic DA neurons.

Functional recovery has been obtained in animal experiments only when the mesencephalic DA-rich grafts had been placed near the denervated target area, i.e., within or directly outside the striatum. This is most probably due to the inability of the grafted DA neurons to extend their axons over a great distance. However, in their ectopic striatal location the grafts can restore only part of the anatomic and functional connections that are characteristic of normal mesostriatal DA neurons. The inability of a graft to reverse a functional deficit in an experimental animal or in a patient with PD might therefore reflect its insufficient integration with host neuronal circuitries. More complete integration would probably require the implantation of grafts into the ventral mesencephalon, where the neurons could receive their normal inputs; on the other hand, this would in turn necessitate a growth of axons sufficient for them to reach the striatum. In a recent study [50], human embryonic DA neurons implanted into the substantia nigra of immunosuppressed rats were observed to grow along the mesostriatal pathway and to give rise to a terminal plexus in the denervated caudate putamen. Although their implications for human-to-human ICG trials are as yet unclear, these results indicate that the activity of presumed growth-inhibiting factors present along the pathway might be overcome under certain conditions.

In all clinical ICG trials in PD performed so far, the embryonic DA neurons have been placed in the caudate nucleus, the putamen, or both. However, also the ventral striatum and especially the nucleus accumbens might be a critical implantation site. In rat experiments, grafts in the nucleus accumbens can increase locomotion [8]. Patients with marked impairments in gait initiation and speed might therefore need grafts in the nucleus accumbens for optimal symptomatic recovery.

There is biochemical evidence that mesencephalic DA neurons also outside the mesostriatal system undergo degeneration in PD, e.g., those projecting to frontal and limbic cortical areas, globus pallidus, and subthalamic nuclei. The DA deficiency in the striatum, which is recognized as the major cause of the motor abnormalities, probably does not account for all the symptoms of PD. Damage to other DA systems may be implicated in the disturbances of motor and cognitive functions as well as of mood; accordingly, restoration of DA transmission by grafts also in nonstriatal areas might be necessary for optimal relief.

Other Approaches

Sources of catecholamine-producing donor tissue other than AM cells and embryonic DA neurons are being explored primarily in animal experiments. Cells from the superior cervical ganglion survive implantation into the striatum, show axonal outgrowth, and alleviate parkinsonian symptoms in MPTP-treated monkeys [37]. Immortalized cell lines such as line PC12 represent a potential source of graft tissue that can ensure a continuous supply of DA, but they are unsuitable for clinical use since they either form tumors or are rejected by the host; however, enclosing them in polymer capsules might prevent both their uncontrolled

growth and their being rejected and make possible their long-term survival [1].

Another exciting strategy consists in implanting cells that have been genetically engineered to synthesize and release dopa or DA (see the chapter by Gage and Fisher, this volume). Fibroblasts and cell lines in which the tyrosine hydroxylase gene has been introduced by infection or transfection can release dopa and/or DA in vitro and in vivo and ameliorate apomorphine-induced rotational asymmetry after implantation into the denervated rat striatum [25, 52]. Much experimental work, however, remains to be done before the clinical usefulness of such cells in PD can be assessed. For example, the ability to extend neurites and form synapses, and the possible functional significance thereof, need to be investigated for each cell type. In addition, the ability of each cell type to reverse parkinsonian deficits must be carefully assessed in animals.

Conclusions

The demonstration that embryonic DA-rich neural grafts can survive and have functional effects in the human parkinsonian brain, as it can in rodents and nonhuman primates, is an important step towards an ICG therapy in PD. However, despite these very encouraging results there exists at present no treatment for PD based on ICG. It is important that patients and their relatives be informed that this research is still at an experimental stage. Clinical ICG trials in PD should be encouraged in centers in which a systematic scientific approach can be adhered to and careful assessment of the patients performed.

Human embryonic mesencephalic tissue currently represents the best material for ICG in PD, but other sources of donor tissue must be explored in parallel, mainly in animal experiments. It is likely that the degree of recovery of individual symptoms will depend on the graft's mechanism of action. Possibly, grafts that release DA or dopa in a diffuse manner ("biologic minipumps") can affect some "simple" behavioral deficits, whereas the reversal of "complex" symptoms will require a synaptic release of DA regulated, at least in part, by the host brain. If so, the choice of tissue for ICG might in the future be based on the pattern of symptoms present in the individual patient. This pattern, probably combined with PET scans to visualize the DA system, may also determine the optimal graft placement. The functional heterogeneity of the DA system in the human striatum is understood only in part. A major objective for studies in nonhuman primates will therefore be to elucidate how grafts placed in different subregions differentially affect various parkinsonian symptoms. Even resorting to many implantation sites will probably not enable the graft-derived DA reinnervation to reach all denervated regions; besides, some of the symptoms might be unrelated to the DA deficit and maximal improvement then achieved only if ICG is combined with other forms of treatment.

In PD, finally, a continuing process of DA neuron degeneration could extend to the grafted cells and damage them. No evidence for such a process has been found; should it nevertheless be seen to take place, a strategy to protect the grafted neurons would have to be developed.

For the development of an ICG therapy in PD, further animal research is necessary but insufficient; since idiopathic PD does not exist in animals, progress in this field will also require clinical trials in patients who are closely monitored before and after transplantation with regard both to functional aspects and graft survival.

Acknowledgements. Our own research reviewed in this chapter was supported by the Swedish MRC (14X-8666), Magnus Bergvalls Stiftelse, Kocks Stiftelse, NHR, and the Medical Faculty, University of Lund. We are most grateful to Gerd Andersson for valuable secretarial help and to Bengt Mattsson for planning the illustrations.

References

1. Aebischer P, Tresco PA, Winn SR, Greene LA, Jaeger CB (1991) Long-term cross-species brain transplantation of a polymer-encapsulated dopamine-secreting cell line. Exp Neurol 111: 269–275
2. Backlund E-O, Granberg P-O, Hamberger B, Knutsson E, Mårtensson A, Sedvall G, Seiger Å, Olson L (1985) Transplantation of adrenal medullary tissue to striatum in parkinsonism. First clinical trials. J Neurosurg 62: 169–173
3. Bankiewicz KS, Plunkett RJ, Jacobowitz DM, Porrino L, Di Porzio U, London WT, Kopin IJ, Oldfield EH (1990) The effect of fetal mesencephalon implants on primate MPTP-induced parkinsonism. Histochemical and behavioural studies. J Neurosurg 72: 231–244
4. Björklund A, Stenevi U (1979) Reconstruction of the nigrostriatal pathway by intracerebral nigral transplants. Brain Res 177: 555–560
5. Bohn MC, Cupit L, Marciano F, Gash DM (1987) Adrenal medulla grafts enhance recovery of striatal dopaminergic fibers. Science 237: 913–916
6. Brown VJ, Dunnett SB (1989) Comparison of adrenal and foetal nigral grafts on drug-induced rotation in rats with 6-OHDA lesions. Exp Brain Res 78: 214–218
7. Brundin P, Nilsson OG, Strecker RE, Lindvall O, Åstedt B, Björklund A (1986) Behavioural effects of human fetal dopamine neurons grafted in a rat model of Parkinson's disease. Exp Brain Res 65: 235–240
8. Brundin P, Strecker RE, Londos E, Björklund A (1987) Dopamine neurons grafted unilaterally to the nucleus accumbens affect drug-induced circling and locomotion. Exp Brain Res 69: 183–194
9. Brundin P, Strecker RE, Widner H, Clarke DJ, Nilsson OG, Åstedt B, Lindvall O, Björklund A (1988) Human fetal dopamine neurons grafted in a rat model of Parkinson's disease: immunological aspects, spontaneous and drug-induced behaviour, and dopamine release. Exp Brain Res 70: 192–208
10. Clarke DJ, Brundin P, Strecker RE, Nilsson OG, Björklund A, Lindvall O (1988) Human fetal dopamine neurons grafted in a rat model of Parkinson's disease: ultrastructural evidence for synapse formation using tyrosine hydroxylase immunocytochemistry. Exp Brain Res 73: 115–126
11. Cunningham LA, Hansen JT, Short MP, Bohn MC (1991) The use of genetically altered astrocytes to provide nerve growth factor to adrenal chromaffin cells grafted into the striatum. Brain Res 561: 192–202
12. Decombe R, Rivot JP, Aunis D, Abrous N, Peschanski M, Herman JP (1990) Importance of catecholamine release for the functional action of intrastriatal implants of adrenal medullary cells: pharmacological analysis and *in vivo* electrochemistry. Exp Neurol 107: 143–153
13. Doucet G, Brundin P, Descarries L, Björklund A (1990) Effect of prior dopamine denervation on survival and fiber outgrowth from intrastriatal fetal mesencephalic grafts. Eur J Neurosci 2: 279–290
14. Dubach M, German DC (1990) Extensive survival of chromaffin cells in adrenal medulla "ribbon" grafts in the monkey neostriatum. Exp Neurol 110: 167–180
15. Dunnett SB (1991) Transplantation of embryonic dopamine neurons: what we know from rats. J Neurol 238: 65–74
16. Dunnett SB, Annett LE (1991) Nigral transplants in primate models of parkinsonism. In: Lindvall O, Björklund A, Widner H (eds) Intracerebral transplantation in movement disorders. Elsevier, Amsterdam, pp 27–51
17. Dunnett SB, Björklund A, Stenevi U, Iversen SD (1981) Behavioural recovery following transplantation of substantia nigra in rats subjected to 6-OHDA lesions of the nigrostriatal pathway: II. Bilateral lesions. Brain Res 229: 457–470
18. Dunnett SB, Whishaw IQ, Rogers DC, Jones GH (1987) Dopamine rich grafts ameliorate whole body motor asymmetry and sensory neglect but not independent limb use in rats with 6-hydroxy-dopamine lesions. Brain Res 415: 63–78
19. Freed CR, Breeze RE, Rosenberg NL, Schneck SA, Wells TH, Barrett JN, Grafton ST, Huang SC, Eidelberg D, Rottenberg DA (1990) Transplantation of human fetal dopamine cells for Parkinson's disease: results at 1 year. Arch Neurol 47: 505–512
20. Freed WJ, Poltorak M, Becker JB (1990) Intracerebral adrenal medulla grafts: a review. Exp Neurol 110: 139–166
21. Goetz CG, Stebbins GT, Klawans HL, Koller WC, Grossman RG, Bakay RAE, Penn RD, United Parkinson Foundation Neural Transplantation Registry (1991) United Parkinson Foundation Neurotransplantation Registry on adrenal medullary transplants: presurgical, and 1- and 2-year follow-up. Neurology 41: 1719–1722
22. Henderson BTH, Clough CG, Hughes RC, Hitchcock ER, Kenny BG (1991) Implantation of human fetal ventral mesencephalon to the right caudate nucleus in advanced Parkinson's disease. Arch Neurol 48: 822–827
23. Hirsch EC, Duyckaerts C, Javoy-Agid F, Hauw J-J, Agid Y (1990) Does adrenal graft enhance recovery of dopaminergic neurons in Parkinson's disease? Ann Neurol 27: 676–682
24. van Horne CG, Mahalik T, Hoffer B, Bygdeman M, Almqvist P, Stieg P, Seiger Å, Olson L, Strömberg I (1990) Behavioural and electrophysiological correlates of human mesencephalic dopaminergic xenograft function in the rat striatum. Brain Res Bull 25: 325–334
25. Horellou P, Brundin P, Kalén P, Mallet J, Björklund A (1990) In vivo release of DOPA and dopamine from genetically engineered cells grafted to the denervated rat striatum. Neuron 5: 393–402
26. Kordower JG, Cochran E, Penn RD, Goetz CG (1991) Putative chromaffin cell survival and enhanced host-derived TH-fiber innervation following a functional adrenal medulla autograft for Parkinson's disease. Ann Neurol 29: 405–412
27. Kordower JH, Fiandaca MS, Notter FD, Hansen JT, Gash DM (1990) NGF-like trophic support from peripheral nerve for grafted rhesus adrenal chromaffin cells. J Neurosurg 73: 418–428
28. Lindvall O, Backlund E-O, Farde L, Sedvall G, Freedman R, Hoffer B, Nobin A, Seiger Å, Olson L (1987) Transplantation in Parkinson's disease: two cases of adrenal medullary grafts to putamen. Ann Neurol 22: 457–468

29. Lindvall O, Rehncrona S, Brundin P, Gustavii B, Åstedt B, Widner H, Lindholm T, Björklund A, Leenders KL, Rothwell JC, Frackowiak R, Marsden CD, Johnels B, Steg G, Freedman R, Hoffer BJ, Seiger Å, Bygdeman M, Strömberg I, Olson L (1989) Human fetal dopamine neurons grafted into the striatum in two patients with severe Parkinson's disease: a detailed account of methodology and a 6 month follow-up. Arch Neurol 46: 615–631

30. Lindvall O, Brundin P, Widner H, Rehncrona S, Gustavii B, Frackowiak R, Leenders KL, Sawle G, Rothwell JC, Marsden CD, Björklund A (1990) Grafts of fetal dopamine neurons survive and improve motor function in Parkinson's disease. Science 247: 574–577

31. Lindvall O, Widner H, Rehncrona S, Brundin P, Odin P, Gustavii B, Frackowiak R, Leenders KL, Sawle G, Rothwell JC, Björklund A, Marsden CD (1992) Transplantation of fetal dopamine neurons in Parkinson's disease: 1-year clinical and neurophysiological observations in two patients with putaminal implants. Ann Neurol 31: 155–165

32. López-Lozano JJ, Bravo G, Brera B, Uría J, Dargallo J, Salmean J, Insausti J, Cerrolaza J, CPH Neural Transplantation Group (1991) Can an analogy be drawn between the clinical evolution of Parkinson's patients who undergo autoimplantation of adrenal medulla and those of fetal ventral mesencephalon transplant recipients? In: Lindvall O, Björklund A, Widner H (eds) Intracerebral transplantation in movement disorders. Elsevier, Amsterdam, pp 87–98

33. Madrazo I, Drucker-Colin R, Diaz V, Martinez-Marta J, Torres C, Becerril JJ (1987) Open microsurgical autograft of adrenal medulla to the right caudate nucleus in Parkinson's disease: a report of two cases. N Engl J Med 316: 831–834

34. Madrazo I, Franco-Bourland R, Ostrosky-Solis F, Aguilera M, Cuevas C, Alvarez F, Magallon E, Zamorano C, Morelos A (1990) Neural transplantation (auto-adrenal, fetal nigral and fetal adrenal) in Parkinson's disease: the Mexican experience. Progr Brain Res 82: 593–602

35. Mandel RJ, Brundin P, Björklund A (1990) The importance of graft placement and task complexity for transplant-induced recovery of simple and complex sensorimotor deficits in dopamine denervated rats. Eur J Neurosci 2: 888–894

36. Molina H, Quiñones R, Alvarez L, Galarraga J, Piedra J, Suárez C, Rachid M, García JC, Perry TL, Santana A, Carmenate H, Macías R, Torres O, Rojas MJ, Córdova F, Muñoz JL (1991) Transplantation of human fetal mesencephalic tissue in caudate nucleus as treatment for Parkinson's disease: the Cuban experience. In: Lindvall O, Björklund A, Widner H (eds) Intracerebral transplantation in movement disorders. Elsevier, Amsterdam, pp 99–110

37. Nakai M, Itakura T, Kamei I, Nakai K, Naka Y, Imai H, Komai N (1990) Autologous transplantation of the superior cervical ganglion into the brain of parkinsonian monkeys. J Neurosurg 72: 92–95

38. Olson L, Backlund E-O, Ebendal T, Freedman R, Hamberger B, Hansson P, Hoffer B, Lindblom U, Meyerson B, Strömberg I, Sydow O, Seiger Å (1991) Intraputaminal infusion of nerve growth factor to support adrenal medullary autografts in Parkinson's disease. One-year follow-up of first clinical trial. Arch Neurol 48: 373–381

39. Otto D, Unsicker K (1990) Basic FGF reverses chemical and morphological deficits in the nigrostriatal system of MPTP treated mice. J Neurosci 10: 1912–1921

40. Perlow MJ, Freed WJ, Hoffer BJ, Seiger Å, Olson L, Wyatt RJ (1979) Brain grafts reduce motor abnormalities produced by destruction of nigrostriatal dopamine system. Science 204: 643–647

41. Plunkett RJ, Bankiewicz KS, Cummins AC, Miletich RS, Schwartz JP, Oldfield EH (1990) Long-term evaluation of hemiparkinsonian monkeys after adrenal autografting or cavitation alone. J Neurosurg 73: 918–926

42. Pezzoli G, Fahn S, Dwork A, Truong DD, de Yebenes JG, Jackson-Lewis V, Herbert J, Cadet JL (1988) Non-chromaffin tissue plus nerve growth factor reduces experimental parkinsonism in aged rats. Brain Res 459: 398–403

43. Sauer H, Brundin P (1991) Effects of cool storage on survival and function of intrastriatal ventral mesencephalic grafts. Restor Neurol Neurosci 2: 123–135

44. Sawle GV, Bloomfield PM, Björklund A, Brooks DJ, Brundin P, Leenders KL, Lindvall O, Marsden CD, Rehncrona S, Widner H, Frackowiak RSJ (1992) Transplantation of fetal dopamine neurons in Parkinson's disease: positron emission tomography [^{18}F]-6-L-fluorodopa studies in two patients with putaminal implants. Ann Neurol 31: 166–173

45. Schwarz SS, Freed WJ (1987) Brain tissue transplantation in neonatal rats prevents a lesion-induced syndrome of adipsia, aphagia and akinesia. Exp Brain Res 65: 449–454

46. Strömberg I, Almqvist P, Bygdeman M, Finger TE, Gerhardt G, Granholm A-C, Mahalik TJ, Seiger Å, Olson L, Hoffer B (1989) Human fetal mesencephalic tissue grafted to dopamine-denervated striatum of athymic rats: Light- and electron-microscopic histochemistry and in vivo chronoamperometric studies. J Neurosci 9: 614–624

47. Strömberg I, Bygdeman M, Goldstein M, Seiger Å, Olson L (1986) Human fetal substantia nigra grafted to the dopamine-denervated striatum of immunosuppressed rats: evidence for functional reinnervation. Neurosci Lett 71: 271–276

48. Strömberg I, Herrera-Marschitz M, Ungerstedt U, Ebendal T, Olson L (1985) Chronic implants of chromaffin tissue into the dopamine-denervated striatum. Effects of NGF on graft survival, fiber growth and rotational behavior. Exp Brain Res 60: 335–349

49. Strömberg I, van Horne C, Bygdeman M, Weiner N, Gerhardt GA (1991) Function of intraventricular human mesencephalic xenografts in immunosuppressed rats: an electrophysiological and neurochemical analysis. Exp Neurol 112: 140–152

50. Wictorin K, Brundin P, Sauer H, Lindvall O, Björklund A (1992) Long distance directed axonal growth from human dopaminergic mesencephalic neuroblasts implanted along the nigrostriatal pathway in 6-hydroxydopamine lesioned adult rats. J Comp Neurol 323: 475–494

51. Widner H, Tetrud J, Rehncrona S, Snow B, Brundin P, Gustavii B, Björklund A, Lindvall O, Langston JW (1992) Bilateral fetal mesencephalic grafting in two patients with parkinsonism induced by 1-methyl-4-phenyl-1,2,3,6-tetrahydropyridine (MPTP). N Engl J Med 327: 1556–1563

52. Wolff JA, Fisher LJ, Xu L, Jinnah HA, Langlais PJ, Iuvone PM, O'Malley KL, Rosenberg MB, Shimohama S, Friedmann T, Gage FH (1989) Grafting fibroblasts genetically modified to produce L-dopa in a rat model of Parkinson disease. Proc Natl Acad Sci USA 86: 9011–9014

Transplantation in Huntington's Disease: Experimental Basis and Clinical Perspectives

A. Björklund and K. Wictorin

Department of Medical Cell Research, Section of Neurobiology, University of Lund, Lund, Sweden

Introduction

Huntington's disease (HD) is an inherited autosomal dominant neurodegenerative disease in the pathogenesis of which a locus on chromosome 4 is thought to play an as yet undetermined role. Atrophy of the striatum, associated with extensive neuronal loss, is the most constant neuropathologic finding, and the extent of striatal atrophy has been correlated with the progression of the disease [21]. Affected patients, in whom the disease usually develops at 35–45 years of age, show a series of symptoms including severe cognitive and emotional disturbances and incapacitating involuntary movements (chorea). The disease generally progresses over 10–20 years, leading directly or indirectly to death (for comprehensive reviews, see [2] and [12]).

There is no naturally occurring model of HD. Coyle and Schwartz [5] and McGeer and McGeer [28] were the first to report that injections of the potent excitatory glutamate analogue kainic acid into the striatum of rats can be used to induce extensive neuronal degeneration without damage to the axons passing through the injected area. Since then, other excitotoxic amino acids such as ibotenic acid and quinolinic acid have been used for the same purpose. Rats with excitotoxic striatal lesions exhibit neuropathologic and neurochemical changes that resemble those seen in the brains of severely affected HD patients. Although such rats do not express choreic symptoms, their motor behavior and cognitive functions are greatly impaired [8, 31, 35]. Many criteria for a good experimental model of the human disease are thus fulfilled. The model can also be used in subhuman primates [11, 18, 19].

Experimental Model

Injections of ibotenic or kainic acid into the head of the caudate-putamen in rats cause over 90%-95% neuronal cell loss in the injected area, accompanied by reactive gliosis and a reduction of the transmitter-related enzymes glutamic acid decarboxylase (GAD) and choline acetyltransferase (ChAT) by 70%–85% [14, 15, 39]. From about 4 weeks af-ter injection there is a progressive atrophy of the neuron-depleted area, resulting in up to 60%–70% reduction in volume and a 50%–55% reduction in weight of the head of the caudate-putamen by 3–4 months [14, 15]. There are signs of neuronal cell loss also in the neocortex and the globus pallidus [17, 32] and the pars reticularis of the substantia nigra [34]. As a consequence of the striatal atrophy, the adjacent lateral ventricle is greatly enlarged. The magnitude of the atrophic changes caused by large doses of ibotenic acid (16–20 µg) is similar to that seen in advanced cases of HD [2].

Implants of Fetal Striatal Primordia

The idea underlying the current intracerebral grafting (ICG) strategy in animals is to restore a striatum-like structure at the damaged site. Striatal primordia are obtained from the developing ganglionic eminences of rat fetuses, as shown in Fig. 1. In our studies we use tissue from E 14 or E 15 donors (embryonic day 14 or 15), in which striatal neurogenesis is at its maximum. After mild trypsinization, the tissue is dispersed into a milky cell suspension. With a microsyringe, we generally inject $4–10 \times 10^5$ cells, corresponding to about one or two striatal primordia, into the lesioned striatum. Alternative procedures, used in other laboratories, have employed older tissues, from E 17–E 19 rat fetuses, implanted as small fragments or larger solid pieces [7, 30, 36].

The cell suspension grafts will grow to reach a final size of about 5–12 mm^3 [14, 15]. As a result, the neuron-depleted atrophic striatum increases in volume from about 30%–50% to about 70%–80% of its normal size. According to Labandeira-Garcia et al. [22], the intrastriatal grafts develop and mature with a time course that is fairly close to that of the normal striatum. The implants increase five- to eightfold in volume over the first 3 weeks, and they appear to have reached their final size and anatomic maturation by 6–8 weeks. Interestingly, the final size of initially similar grafts is smaller when implanted into the non-lesioned striatum [22] or into other brain regions such as the globus pallidus, the substantia nigra, or the neocortex [17] than in the

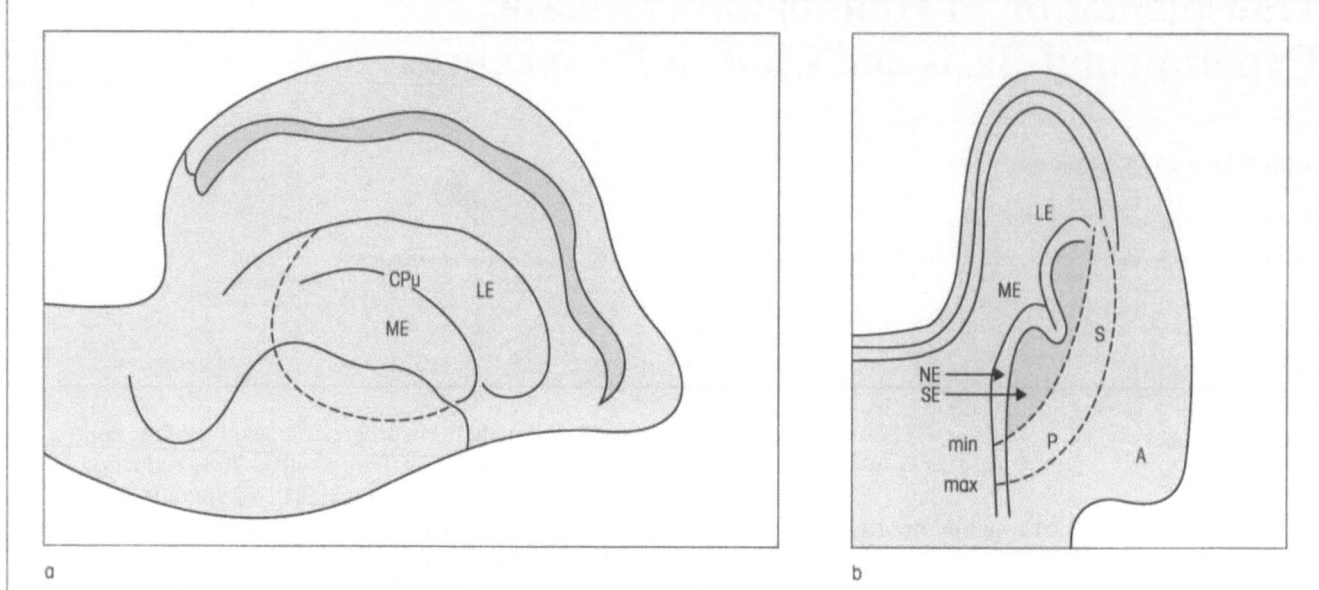

Fig. 1 a, b. *Schematic drawing of the E 14 rat embryonic forebrain and the regions dissected for the preparation of striatal cell suspensions.* **a** *Medial view of the lateral ventricle wall with the two elevations (medial,* **ME***, and lateral,* **LE***) of the ganglionic eminences, which constitute the anlage for the caudate-putamen (**CPu**). The* **dashed line** *approximately indicates the region that is dissected.* **b** *Coronal section through the cen-* *ter of the region shown in* **a***. Here the* **dashed lines** *show the approximate minimal (**min**) and maximal (**max**) extents, respectively, of the dissections. The lateral ventricular wall consists of a neuroepithelium (**NE**), a subependymal layer (**SE**), and the anlages for striatum (**S**), pallidum (**P**), and amygdala (**A**), as well as lateral cortical regions. (Modified from [49])*

excitotoxin-lesioned striatum. This implies that trophic interactions between the host brain environment and the graft play an important role in the growth and maturation of the neuroblasts and neuroepithelial stem cells contained in the striatal cell suspension.

Intrinsic Organization of the Striatal Grafts

The striatal grafts have been shown to contain many of the neuron types characteristic for the intact neostriatum, such as GABA-ergic and cholinergic neurons, and they express several of the characteristic neuropeptides such as met-enkephalin, substance P, somatostatin, and neuropeptide Y [see 4, 10, 17, 42]. Dopamine and opiate receptor autoradiography, in combination with calbindin, met-enkephalin, and acetylcholinesterase staining, has provided evidence that the two histochemical compartments, patch and matrix, normally present in the neostriatum also develop in the striatal grafts [10, 17, 25, 49]. Immunohistochemistry using antibodies to characteristic striatal markers such as DARPP-32 (a dopamine- and adenosine 3',5'-monophosphate-regulated phosphoprotein with a molecular weight of 32 kDa) and calbindin indicates that the striatal grafts have a heterogeneous composition. As shown in Fig. 2, the DARPP-32-pos-

itive striatal compartment is confined to patches that constitute one-third to one-half of the total cross-sectional graft area [10, 49]. The remaining areas are likely to represent other basal forebrain regions, such as cortex, amygdala, or pallidum, known to be generated from the ganglionic eminence or adjacent regions during normal brain development (see Fig. 1).

Biochemical Markers of Striatal Graft Maturation and Function

Biochemical assays of GAD and ChAT enzyme activity [15] have shown a substantial recovery of GABA and acetylcholine synthesis in the grafted striatum at 20 weeks, but not at 3 weeks, after transplantation. Consistent with this, measurements of extracellular GABA overflow by intracerebral microdialysis [3] have shown that striatal GABA release, which is markedly depressed in the ibotenic-acid-lesioned striatum, is normalized by the striatal grafts. A graft-induced recovery of GAD activity [15] and GABA release [41] was observed also in the globus pallidus.

In rats with unilateral striatal lesions [14], measurement of local cerebral metabolism by means of the autoradiographic method of Sokoloff [44] have demonstrated a 60%

Fig. 2 a, b. *Microphotographs of two adjacent sections through the center of an intrastriatal striatal transplant showing* **a** *DARPP-32-immunoreactive cells and* **b** *tyrosine-hydroxylase-positive (TH-positive) host afferents. The DARPP-32-positive cells are organized in distinct striatum-like patches (**P** regions) separated by nonpatch areas (**NP** regions) with virtually no densely DARPP-32-immunoreactive elements. The TH-positive host afferents provide a dense and specific innervation of the P regions.* **CC**, *corpus callosum;* **H**, *host;* **T**, *transplant. Scale bars, 250 μm. (Modified from [49]).*

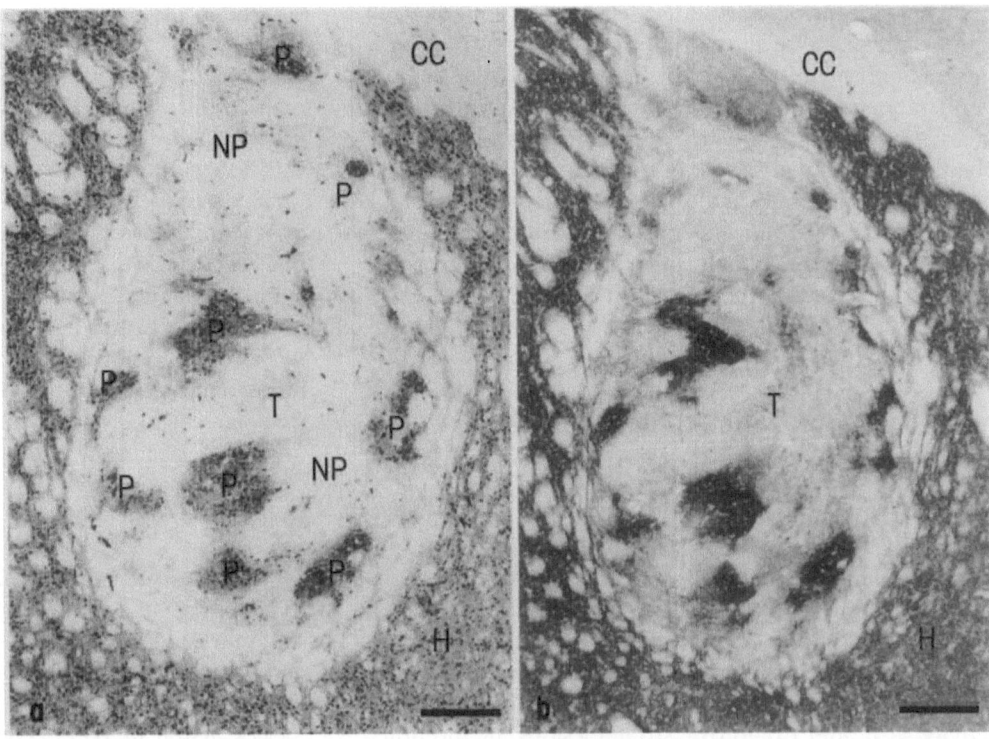

Fig. 3. **a** *The major fiber pathways that interconnect the striatal output structures.* **CPu**, *caudate-putamen;* **GP**, *globus pallidus;* **SUT**, *subthalamic nucleus;* **SNc**, *substantia nigra, pars compacta;* **SNr**, *substantia nigra, pars reticularis;* **Coll. sup.**, *colliculus superior.* **b, c** *Schematic diagrams of local [14C]2-deoxy-d-glucose utilization in major striatal output areas after a striatal lesion induced by ibotenic acid (**gray area** in **b**) and after such a lesion followed by transplantation of striatal tissue (**Trpl** in **c**). The values in **b** and **c** express the increase in glucose utilization from values in intact control animals, and the **asterisks** in **c** mark the structures in which a significant reduction, i. e., normalization, was achieved after transplantation. (Data from [14])*

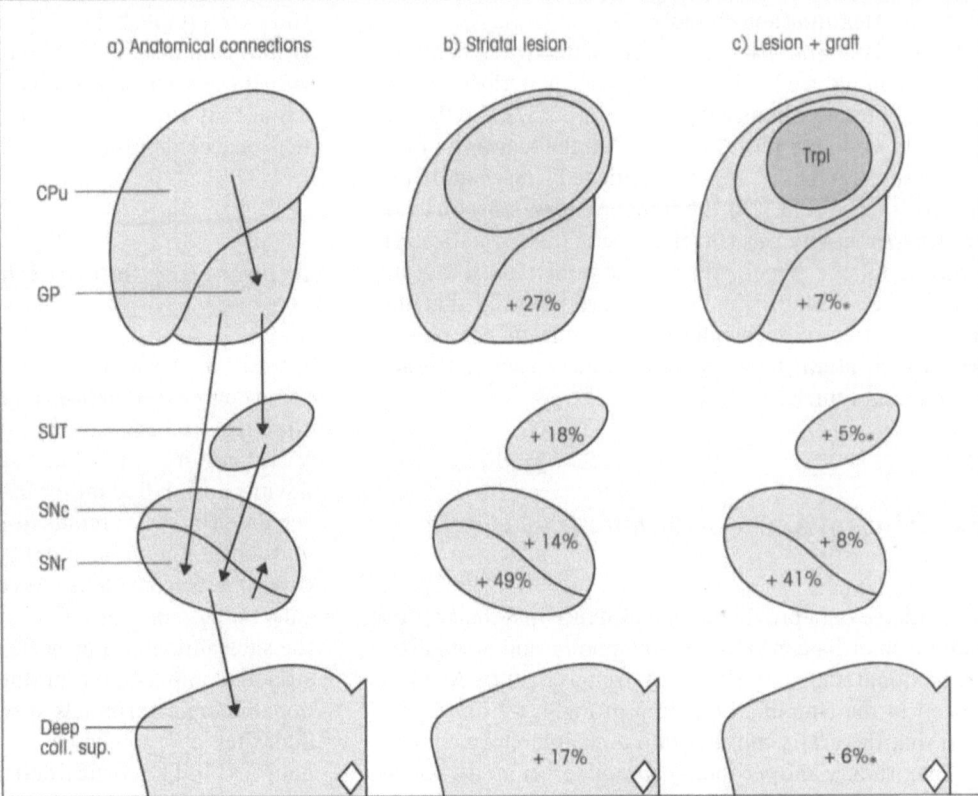

reduction in glucose utilization throughout the lesioned striatum. In contrast, the contralateral striatum displayed a 20%–30% increase in mean glucose utilization. All major primary and secondary striatal projection areas (Fig. 3) showed significant unilateral or bilateral increases in metabolic rates, the strongest increases being seen in the pars reticularis of the substantia nigra, the globus pallidus, the subthalamic nucleus, and the deep layers of the superior colliculus. Striatal implants were found to exhibit a significant glucose utilization rate amounting to about 70% of that in the intact control neostriatum. The striatal graft did not significantly increase glucose utilization in the surrounding (lesioned or spared) areas of the host striatum, but the hypermetabolic responses seen in the striatal projection areas in lesioned but nongrafted rats were normalized by the implant, ipsilaterally in the globus pallidus and subthalamic nucleus, and bilaterally in the deep superior colliculi (asterisks in Fig. 3). A significant transplant-induced effect was seen also in the functionally associated ventral tegmental area and nucleus accumbens.

Amelioration of Lesion-Induced Behavioral Deficits

These metabolic data are consistent with the view that large striatal lesions (such as those seen in HD) remove a major inhibitory, probably largely GABA-ergic, control of downstream extrapyramidal motor centers. In HD, such disinhibition is thought to account for the choreic movements. In the rat, the best behavioral correlate is the locomotor hyperactivity seen after excitotoxic striatal lesions. In addition, the lesions induce long-lasting deficits in skilled motor functions, resulting in defective paw use in the rat, as well as impairment of learning and memory.

Intrastriatal grafts are remarkably effective in counteracting lesion-induced behavioral deficits: hyperlocomotion is largely or totally abolished [6, 7, 14, 16, 36, 37], and the impairments in skilled paw use [9] and in the learning of delayed-response tasks [7, 16] are significantly lessened. In the study by Isacson et al. [14], the compensatory effect on locomotor hyperactivity was correlated with the normalization of the metabolic hyperactivity in several striatal output structures, and Sanberg et al. [37] have reported that the functional effect is seen only when the grafts are placed within the striatum, not when they are placed within the adjacent lateral ventricle.

Mechanisms of Action of the Intrastriatal Grafts

The available data provide strong evidence that the grafted striatal primordia can substantially modify, and normalize, the functional state of the lesioned striatal circuitry. As summarized in the simplified diagram in Fig. 4, we have proposed that the grafts can reinstate tonic inhibitory control over the primary and secondary striatal target areas, above all the globus pallidus, subthalamic nucleus, and substantia nigra. In the intact animal, these control functions are mediated by the striatal efferent neurons, which project to the globus pallidus and substantia nigra. These neurons are, in turn, regulated by major inputs, mainly from the substantia nigra, frontoparietal cortex, and intralaminar thalamic nuclei.

The functional graft-host interaction proposed in Fig. 4 assumes the existence of a functional connection between the striatal graft and the striatal output structures. The increased glucose utilization seen in the primary striatal target areas, namely the globus pallidus and the substantia nigra, in rats with striatal excitotoxic lesions shows that the caudate-putamen normally exerts an inhibitory (probably GABA-ergic) tonic control over the functional activity of these output structures. Mogenson and Nielsen [29] have shown that locomotor activity can be modified by the direct administration into the globus pallidus of drugs that act on GABA receptors. It is conceivable, therefore, that the effects of intrastriatal grafts on metabolic and motor hyperactivity in ibotenic-acid-lesioned rats are mediated via the release of GABA. This view is supported by the above-mentioned observations [15, 41] of significant graft-induced increases in GAD activity and GABA overflow in the globus pallidus.

Graft-derived GABA release could be of a diffuse, neurohumoral nature. However, there is considerable neuroanatomic evidence that the medium-sized densely spiny neurons within striatal grafts, which are likely to be GABA-ergic, project out of the transplant. By means of cross-species neural markers (Fig. 5a) and anterograde axonal tracers (Fig. 5b), these efferent axons have been traced along the myelinated fascicles of the internal capsule and shown to establish direct synaptic connections with the host globus pallidus [49–52] and to a minor extent probably also with the host substantia nigra [50]. GABA released from the axons may thus be able to act directly on the denervated neuronal elements in the pallidum.

Afferent Regulation of the Grafted Neurons

Intrastriatal striatal grafts may depend for their effects on some degree of functional integration with the host striatal circuitry, as is suggested by their acting not only on metabolic and motor activity but also on complex conditioned behaviors and skilled motor tasks. Normal striatal function is regulated by major inputs from mainly the cortex, thalamus, and substantia nigra, and the grafts have been shown to receive inputs from all three systems. As illustrated schematically in Fig. 6 (see also Fig. 2), the dopaminergic input from the substantia nigra projects densely and selectively to the striatal compartment of the grafts [32, 49], where the dopaminergic terminals form synaptic contacts with the dendrites and spines of the medium-sized densely spiny neurons [4]. The cortical and thalamic afferents, by contrast, innervate both the striatal and nonstriatal graft compartments, mainly in the peripheral areas [46, 47, 53, 54]. There is both electron microscopic and electrophysiologic evidence that the cortical and thalamic host afferents form functional synaptic contacts with the grafted neurons [33, 48, 53, 55].

Host afferents may thus participate in the regulation of

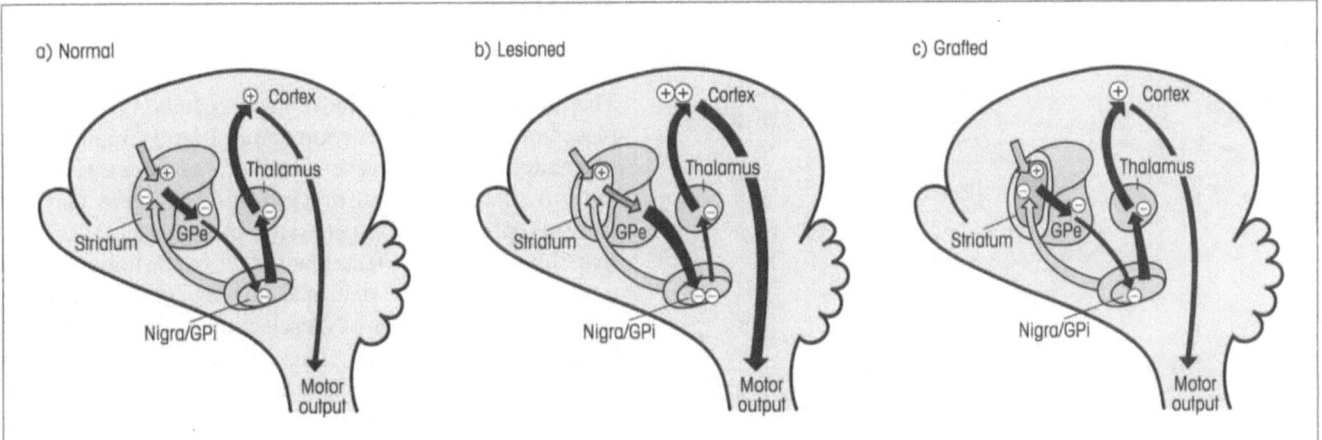

Fig. 4 a–c. *Proposed model of striatal graft function. The drawings show the efferent projections from the striatum and from its related output structures in intact control animals (**a**) and the proposed functional changes induced by a striatal lesion caused by ibotenic acid (**b**) and by such a lesion followed by striatal transplantation (**c**).* **a** *A large portion of the striatal output neurons project to the globus pallidus (**GPe, GPi**, globus pallidus, external segment and internal segment), and the pallidal neurons project to the pars reticularis of the substantia nigra (indirect pathway); other striatal neurons project directly to the substantia nigra (direct pathway). Since the indirect pathway appears to be the one most relevant in the present context, it is the only one included in the drawings; like the downstream nigrothalamocortical output pathways, it is shown* with **black arrows**. *The striatum is under the control of many afferent systems, of which the cortical (**blue arrow**) and the nigral (**green arrow**) are included in the drawings.* **b** *In rats with striatal lesions caused by ibotenic acid (**gray area**), the globus pallidus has lost a large proportion of the inhibitory input from the striatum; the resulting increased activity in the pallidonigral neurons eventually manifests itself as an increased motor output.* **c** *It is proposed that in rats with striatal lesions (**gray area**) and subsequent transplantations (**pink area**) the grafts have reinstated some of the inhibitory striatal influence over the pallidal neurons; the net result is a partly normalized motor output. In addition, the host cortical and nigral afferents have innervated parts of the transplants and can influence and control the activity of the grafted neurons*

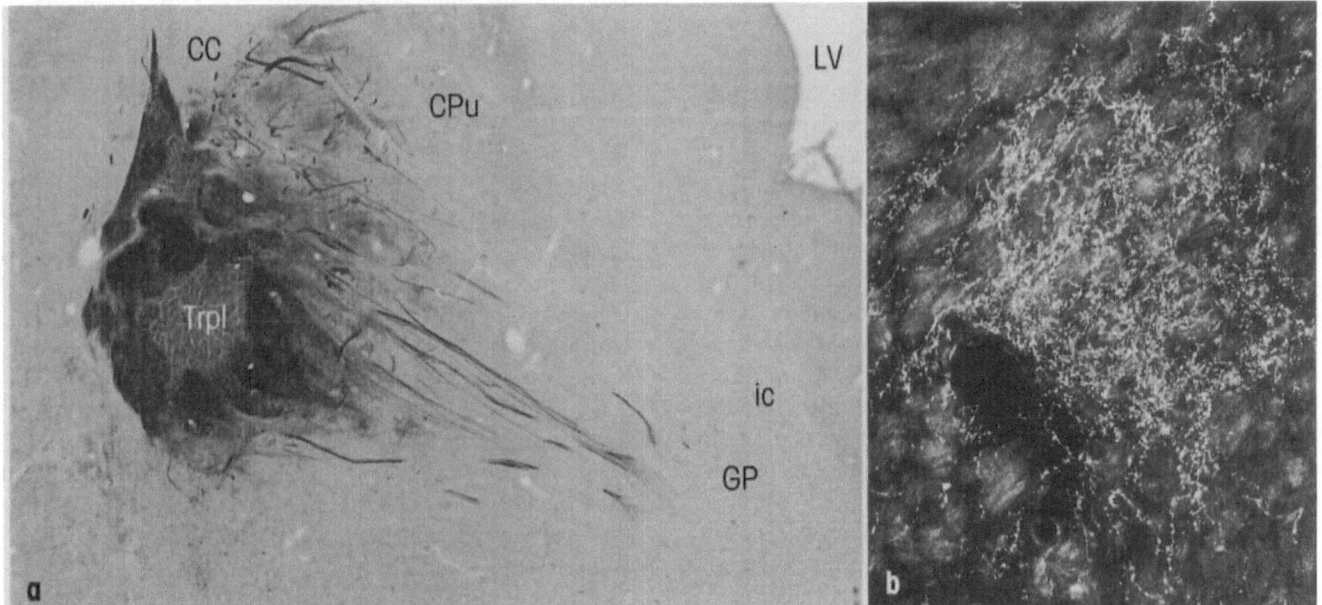

Fig. 5 a, b. *Microphotographs illustrating the efferent axonal projections from the grafts to the host brain. In the sagittal section shown in **a**, mouse fetal striatal tissue has been transplanted into the striatum of an adult rat with a lesion caused by ibotenic acid (IA), and the transplant (**Trpl**) and graft-derived fibers have been detected immunohistochemically with the mouse neuron-specific antiserum M6. Note the dense fascicles of fibers projecting caudally from the Trpl into the rostral globus pallidus (**GP**). In **b**, graft-derived fibers are shown to branch into a terminal* network in the host globus pallidus (**GP**). In this animal with an IA lesion and a subsequent fetal graft, an anterograde tracer (Phaseolus vulgaris leukoagglutinin, PHA-L) was injected several months later into the transplant. Thus, labeled axons could be followed from the transplant into the host brain, where a terminal network was demonstrated in the GP. **CC**, corpus callosum; **CPu**, caudate-putamen; **ic**, internal capsule; **LV**, lateral ventricle. (Modified from [50, 52])

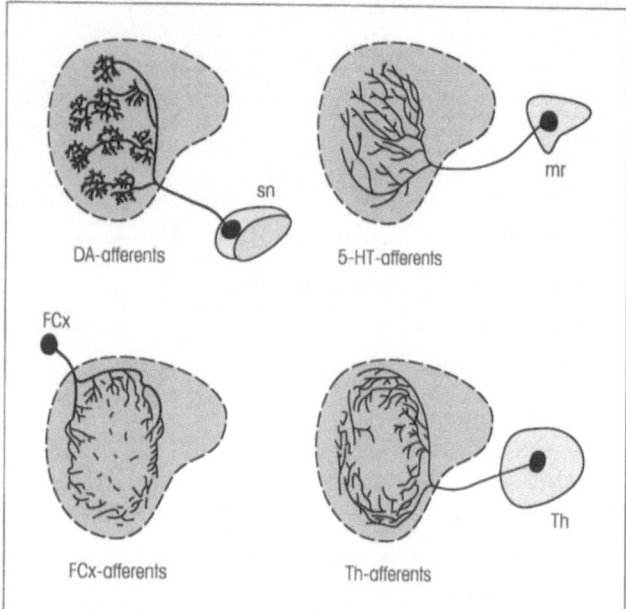

Fig. 6. *Schematic representation of the different patterns of afferent innervation of the striatal transplants provided by various host nuclei. The dopaminergic (**DA**) afferents from the substantia nigra (**sn**) form dense patches of terminals in the striatum-like regions throughout the implants, and the serotoninergic (**5-HT**) afferents from the mesencephalic raphe (**mr**) also reach densities comparable to normal ones within large areas of the implants. Frontal cortical (**FCx**) or thalamic (**Th**) afferents provide a relatively dense innervation, mainly in the more peripheral graft regions*

Trophic Effects of Striatal Transplants

The research discussed above has focused on neuronal replacement and reconstruction of the striatal circuitry in the rat model of HD. However, in other experimental models there are data suggesting that intracerebral grafts may protect from progressive degenerative changes. In several systems, fetal CNS tissue transplants have been shown to counteract lesion-induced neuronal atrophy or the axotomy-induced death of neurons projecting to or through the lesioned area [1, 40, 43]. These trophic-like effects may derive, at least in part, from the nonneuronal (glial) constituents of the implanted tissue. Thus, in experiments on cortical lesions, Kesslak et al. [20] have shown that grafts of fetal cortical tissue can reduce the behavioral consequences of frontal cortical lesions in adult rats and that a similar effect can be exerted also by implants of cultured astrocytes.

Whether striatal grafts can counteract primary or secondary degenerative changes induced by a progressive striatal damage such as is present in HD is still unclear. Tulipan et al. [45] have reported that striatal grafts can reduce the acute damage induced by an excitotoxic lesion, and Schumacher et al. [38] have recently reported that the juxtastriatal implantation of genetically engineered fibroblasts secreting nerve growth factor (NGF) can provide protection against a subsequent injection of quisqualic or quinolinic acid. Even though the relevance of these models for HD – a progressive and genetically determined degenerative process – remains uncertain, the possibility of obtaining neuroprotective effects by implants of fetal CNS tissue, glial cells, or genetically engineered cells deserves to be explored further.

Studies in Primates

The data summarized so far have all been obtained in rodents. In the perspective of clinical applications, studies in nonhuman primates are clearly needed in order to assess the validity of neural ICG in a model that is closer to man. The conclusions that can be drawn from studies in the rat are limited by its striatum's being anatomically and functionally less complex than that of humans. The disturbances in motor function induced by striatal lesions in rodents are thus far less severe than those seen in patients with HD. Moreover, the human striatum is about 200 times larger than the rat's and thus presents a greater challenge for any replacement strategy.

Initial experiments performed by Isacson et al. [11, 18, 19] indicate that the motor deficits induced by striatal excitotoxic lesions in monkeys resemble more closely the symptoms seen in patients with HD. In particular, the abnormal movements and dyskinesias observed after the administration of the dopamine receptor agonist apomorphine bear resemblance to the choreic manifestations of HD [11]. The dyskinesias induced by apomorphine in monkeys with exci-

striatal graft function. The nigrostriatal dopaminergic afferents, in particular, are known to exert a profound permissive influence on striatal functions in the intact animal; several lines of evidence indicate that this regulatory mechanism is present also in striatal grafts. Dunnett et al. [9] and Norman et al. [30], observing the drug-induced turning behavior in rats with unilateral lesions and grafts, have shown that intrastriatal striatal grafts can counteract the motor asymmetry induced by either direct (apomorphine) or indirect (amphetamine) dopamine receptor agonists. More direct evidence for a direct dopaminergic control of the grafted striatal neurons has come from studies using the expression of the Fos oncogene protein (i.e., the product of the immediate-early c-*fos* gene) as a cellular marker for host dopaminergic influences over the grafted neurons [26, 27]. The results show that direct or indirect dopamine receptor activation induces Fos expression in a subpopulation of grafted striatal neurons similar to that seen in the intact striatum, this effect being dependent on the integrity of the host dopaminergic input. In combination with other neuroanatomic and behavioral observations, these data provide compelling evidence that all the elements of a functional nigrostriatopallidal circuitry may be established in the striatal grafts.

totoxic striatal damage were reported to be stable over time and to correlate in severity with the size of the lesions. Isacson et al. [18, 19] have reported on five immunosuppressed baboons in which cross-species grafts of striatal tissue from fetal rats were performed into the lesioned striatal area. All five animals showed a gradual, 60%–80%, reduction in apomorphine-induced dyskinesia scores within 7–10 weeks after grafting. In two monkeys, immunosuppression was discontinued, with reappearance of the symptoms as the grafts were rejected.

Clinical Perspectives

The new strategy of neural ICG has been explored mainly in patients with Parkinson's disease (PD). Accumulating data from ongoing trials indicate that human fetal tissue from the ventral mesencephalon can survive ICG and improve motor functions in patients with severe PD (for recent reviews, see [23, 24]). Furthermore, this approach seems to entail no hazard to the patients.

The experience gained so far might be thought to justify a similar approach in patients with HD. However, caution is required. First, the use of human embryonic tissue raises ethical problems, discussed for instance in [13]. Although human embryonic CNS tissue is currently the only possible source of tissue for transplantation in neurodegenerative disorders, efforts are being made to develop alternatives, e. g., genetically modified cells or immortalized cell lines; these efforts must be pursued. The procurement of embryonic human CNS tissue is also attended with practical problems: the tissue obtained from a single fetus may not be enough, and precise identification and dissection of the striatal primordia must be achieved in spite of the available embryonic forebrains' often being severely disrupted; preclinical experimental trials will have to ensure that the criteria for identifying the striatal primordia are sufficiently reliable.

Possibly, the rat excitotoxin model is not a good experimental model for HD, and thus the results obtained so far in animals might be irrelevant to the human disease. In the rat model, the degeneration of the striatum occurs very rapidly, whereas in HD it is gradual. Besides, it is not known whether the disease process involved in human HD may also affect any implanted neurons; therefore, noninvasive techniques for assessing graft survival, e. g., positron emission tomography or magnetic resonance imaging, should be an essential part of clinical ICG trials.

In spite of the many problems that remain to be solved, there are at least two strong arguments in favor of limited and well-controlled clinical trials of neural ICG in HD. First, there is at present no effective treatment for this severe and fatal disorder. Second, the experience in PD has so far not revealed any serious complications or adverse effects of the ICG of embryonic tissue.

Undoubtedly, more experiments in primates are needed in order to establish the optimal technical prerequisites for neural ICG in the larger and more complex primate brain. The study of excitotoxic striatal lesions in monkeys, as performed by Isacson et al. [11, 18, 19], promises to be highly useful for that purpose.

References

1. Bregman B, Reier PJ (1986) Neural tissue transplants rescue axotomized rubrospinal cells from retrograde death. J Comp Neurol 244: 86–95
2. Bruyn GW (1968) Huntington's chorea, historical, clinical and laboratory synopsis. In: Vinken PJ, Bruyn GW (eds) Handbook of clinical neurology, vol 6, pp 298–378, North-Holland Publ., Amsterdam
3. Campbell K, Kalén P, Wictorin K, Lundberg C, Mandel RM, Björklund A (1993) Characterization of GABA release from intrastriatal striatal transplants: dependence on host-derived afferents. Neuroscience (in press)
4. Clarke DJ, Dunnett SB, Isacson O, Sirinathsinghji DJS, Björklund A (1988) Striatal grafts in rats with unilateral neostriatal lesions: I. Ultrastructural evidence of afferent synaptic inputs from the host nigrostriatal pathway. Neuroscience 24: 791–801
5. Coyle JT, Schwartz R (1976) Lesion of striatal neurones with kainic acid provides a model for Huntington's chorea. Nature 263: 244–246
6. Deckel AW, Robinson RG, Coyle JT, Sanberg PR (1983) Reversal of longterm locomotor abnormalities in the kainic acid model of Huntington's disease by day 18 fetal striatal implants. Eur J Pharmacol 93: 287–288
7. Deckel AW, Moran TH, Coyle JT, Sanberg PR, Robinson RG (1986) Anatomical predictors of behavioral recovery following striatal transplants. Brain Res 365: 249–258
8. Dunnett SB, Iversen SD (1981) Learning impairments following selective kainic acid-induced lesions within the neostriatum of rats. Behav Brain Res 2: 189–209
9. Dunnett SB, Isacson O, Sirinathsinghji DJS, Clarke DJ, Björklund A (1988) Striatal grafts in rats with unilateral neostriatal lesions: recovery from dopamine dependent asymmetry and deficits in skilled paw reaching. Neuroscience 24: 813–820
10. Graybiel AM, Liu FC, Dunnett SB (1989) Intrastriatal grafts derived from fetal striatal primordia: I. Phenotopy and modular organization. J Neurosci 9: 3250–3271
11. Hantraye P, Riche D, Maziere M, Isacson O (1990) An experimental primate model for Huntington's disease: anatomical and behavioural studies of unilateral excitotoxic lesions of the caudate-putamen in the baboon. Exp Neurol 108: 91–104
12. Harper PS (ed) (1991) Huntington's disease. Major problems in neurology, vol 22. Saunders, London
13. Hoffer BJ, Olson L (1991) Ethical issues in brain-cell transplantation. Trends Neurosci 14: 415–418
14. Isacson O, Brundin P, Kelly PAT, Gage FH, Björklund A (1984) Functional neuronal replacement by grafted neurons in the ibotenic acid-lesioned striatum. Nature 311: 458–460
15. Isacson O, Brundin P, Gage FH, Björklund A (1985) Neural grafting in a rat model of Huntington's disease. Progressive neurochemical changes after neostriatal ibotenate lesions and striatal tissue grafting. Neuroscience 16: 799–817
16. Isacson O, Dunnett SB, Björklund A (1986) Graft-induced behavioural recovery in an animal model of Huntington's disease. Proc Natl Acad Sci USA 83: 2728–2732
17. Isacson O, Dawbarn D, Brundin P, Gage FH, Emson PC, Björklund A (1987) Neural grafting in a rat model of Huntington's disease: striosomal-like organization of striatal grafts as revealed by immunocytochemistry and receptor autoradiography. Neuroscience 22: 481–497

18. Isacson O, Riche D, Hantraye P, Sofroniew MV, Maziere M (1989) A primate model of Huntington's disease: cross-species implantation of striatal precursor cells to the excitotoxically lesioned baboon caudate-putamen. Exp Brain Res 75: 213–220

19. Isacson O, Hantraye P, Riche D, Schumacher JM, Mazière M (1991) The relationship between symptoms and functional anatomy in the chronic neurodegenerative diseases: from pharmacological to biological replacement therapy in Huntington's disease. In: Lindvall O, Björklund O, Widner H (eds) Intracerebral transplantation in movement disorders. Elsevier, Amsterdam, pp 245–258

20. Kesslak JP, Nieto-Sampedro M, Globus J, Cotman CW (1986) Transplants of purified astrocytes promote behavioral recovery after frontal cortex ablation. Exp Neurol 92: 377–390

21. Kuhl DE, Phelps ME, Markham C, Winter J, Metter J, Riege W (1982) Cerebral metabolism and atrophy in Huntington's disease determined by ^{18}FDG and computed tomographic scan. Ann Neurol 12: 425–434

22. Labandeira-Garcia JL, Wictorin K, Cunningham Jr ET, Björklund A (1991) Development of intrastriatal striatal grafts and their afferent innervation from the host. Neuroscience 42: 407–426

23. Lindvall O (1989) Transplantation into the human brain: present status and future possibilities. J Neurol Neurosurg Psychiatry [Suppl]: 39–54

24. Lindvall O (1991) Prospect of transplantation in human neurodegenerative diseases. Trends Neurosci 14: 376–384

25. Liu F-C, Graybiel AM, Dunnett SB, Baughman RW (1990) Intrastriatal grafts derived from fetal striatal primordia: II. Compartmental alignment of cholinergic and dopaminergic systems. J Comp Neurol 295: 1–15

26. Liu FC, Dunnett SB, Robertson HA, Graybiel AM (1991) Intrastriatal grafts derived from fetal striatal primordia: III. Introduction of modular patterns of Fos-like immunoreactivity by cocaine. Exp Brain Res 85: 501–506

27. Mandel RJ, Wictorin K, Cenci MA, Björklund A (1992) Fos expression in intrastriatal grafts: regulation by host dopaminergic afferents. Brain Res 583: 207–215

28. McGeer EG, McGeer PL (1976) Duplication of biochemical changes of Huntington's chorea by intrastriatal injection of glutamic and kainic acids. Nature 263: 517–519

29. Mogenson GJ, Nielsen MA (1983) Evidence that an accumbens to subpallidal GABAergic projection contributes to locomotor activity. Brain Res Bull 11: 309–314

30. Norman AB, Giordano M, Sanberg PR (1989) Fetal striatal tissue grafts into excitotoxin-lesioned striatum: pharmacological and behavioural aspects. Pharmacol Biochem Behav 34: 139–147

31. Pisa M, Sanberg PR, Fibiger HC (1981) Striatal injections of kainic acid selectively impair serial memory performance in the rat. Exp Neurol 74: 633–653

32. Pritzel M, Isacson O, Brundin P, Wiklund L, Björklund A (1986) Afferent and efferent connections of striatal grafts implanted into the ibotenic acid lesioned neostriatum in adult rats. Exp Brain Res 65: 112–126

33. Rutherford A, Garcia-Munoz M, Dunnett SB, Arbuthnott GW (1987) Electrophysiological demonstration of host cortical inputs to striatal grafts. Neurosci Lett 83: 275–281

34. Saji M, Reis DJ (1987) Delayed transneuronal death of substantia nigra neurons prevented by gamma-aminobutyric acid agonist. Science 235: 66–69

35. Sanberg PR, Fibiger HC (1979) Body weight, feeding and drinking behaviors in rats with kainic acid lesions of the striatal neurons: with a note on body weight smyptomatology in Huntington's disease. Exp Neurol 66: 444–466

36. Sanberg PR, Henault MA, Deckel AW (1986) Locomotor hyperactivity: effects of multiple striatal transplants in an animal model of Huntington's disease. Pharmacol Biochem Behav 25 [Suppl]: 297–301

37. Sanberg PR, Giordano M, Henault MA, Nash DR, Ragozzino ME, Hagenmayer-Houser SH (1989) Intraparenchymal striatal transplants required for maintenance of behavioural recovery in an animal model of Huntington's disease. J Neural Transpl 1: 23–31

38. Schumacher JM, Short MP, Hyman BT, Breakefield XO, Isacson O (1991) Intracerebral implantation of nerve growth factor-producing fibroblasts protects striatum against neurotoxic levels of excitatory amino acids. Neuroscience 45: 561–570

39. Schwartz R, Hökfelt T, Fuxe K, Jonsson G, Goldstein M, Terenius L (1979) Ibotenic acid-induced neuronal degeneration: a morphological and neurochemical study. Exp Brain Res 37: 199–216

40. Sievers J, Hausmann B, Berry M (1989) Fetal brain grafts rescue adult retinal ganglion cells from axotomy-induced cell death. J Comp Neurol 281: 467–478

41. Sirinathsinghji DJS, Dunnett SB, Isacson O, Clarke DJ, Kendrick K, Björklund A (1988) Striatal grafts in rats with unilateral neostriatal lesions: II. In vivo monitoring of GABA release in globus pallidus and substantia nigra. Neuroscience 24: 803–811

42. Sirinathsinghji DJS, Morris BJ, Wisden W, Northrop A, Hunt SP, Dunnett SB (1990) Gene expression in striatal grafts: I. Cellular localization of neurotransmitter mRNAs. Neuroscience 34: 675–686

43. Sofroniew MV, Isacson O, Björklund A (1986) Cortical grafts prevent atrophy of cholinergic basal nucleus neurons induced by excitotoxic cortical damage. Brain Res 378: 409–415

44. Sokoloff L (1977) Relation between physiological function and energy metabolism in the central nervous system. J Neurochem 29: 13–26

45. Tulipan N, Huang S, Whetsell WO, Allen GS (1986) Neonatal striatal grafts prevent lethal syndrome produced by bilateral intrastriatal injection of kainic acid. Brain Res 377: 163–167

46. Wictorin K, Isacson O, Fischer W, Nithias FH, Peschanski M, Björklund A (1988) Connectivity of striatal grafts implanted into the ibotenic acid lesioned striatum: I. Subcortical afferents. Neuroscience 27: 547–562

47. Wictorin K, Björklund A (1989) Connectivity of striatal grafts implanted into the ibotenic acid lesioned striatum: II. Cortical afferents. Neuroscience 30: 297–311

48. Wictorin K, Clarke DJ, Bolam JP, Björklund A (1989) Host corticostriatal fibres establish synaptic connections with grafts striatal neurons in the ibotenic acid lesioned striatum. Eur J Neurosci 1: 189–195

49. Wictorin K, Ouimet CC, Björklund A (1989) Intrinsic organization and connectivity of intrastriatal striatal transplants in rats as revealed by DARPP-32 immunohistochemistry: specificity of connections with the lesioned host brain. Eur J Neurosci 1: 690–701

50. Wictorin K, Simerly RB, Isacson O, Swanson LW, Björklund A (1989) Connectivity of striatal grafts implanted into the ibotenic acid lesioned striatum: III. Efferent projecting graft neurons and their relation to host afferents with the grafts. Neuroscience 30: 313–330

51. Wictorin K, Clarke DJ, Bolam JP, Björklund A (1990) Fetal striatal neurons grafted into the ibotenate lesioned striatum: efferent projections and synaptic contacts in the host globus pallidus. Neuroscience 37: 301–315

52. Wictorin K, Lagenaur CF, Lund RD, Björklund A (1991) Efferent projections to the host brain from intrastriatal striatal mouse-to-rat grafts: time-course and tissue-type specificity as revealed by a mouse specific neuronal marker. Eur J Neurosci 3: 86–101

53. Xu ZC, Wilson CJ, Emson PC (1989) Restoration of the corticostriatal projection in rat neostriatal grafts: electron microscopic analysis. Neuroscience 29: 539–550

54. Xu ZC, Wilson CJ, Emson PC (1990) Restoration of thalamostriatal projections in rat neostriatal grafts: an electron microscopic analysis. J Comp Neurol 303: 2–14

55. Xu ZC, Wilson CJ, Emson PC (1991) Synaptic potentials evoked in spiny neurons in rat neurostriatal grafts by cortical and thalamic stimulation. J Neurophysiol 65: 477–493

Neural Transplantation in Dementia

S. B. Dunnett

Department of Experimental Psychology, University of Cambridge, Cambridge, UK

Common Terminology in Research on Alzheimer's Disease

Senile dementia	A class of diseases of old age, leading to progressive functional deterioration of cognition, attention, learning, and memory.
Alzheimer's disease (AD)	A neurodegenerative disease that is the commonest cause of dementia. Its diagnosis is based on the presence post mortem of specific neuropathologic hallmarks: neurofibrillary tangles and senile plaques in the neocortex and hippocampus.
Senile dementia of the Alzheimer type (SDAT)	Because a final diagnosis of Alzheimer's disease can only be made post mortem, patients whose dementia is characteristic of AD should in life strictly be diagnosed as having SDAT.
Neurofibrillary tangles (NFTs)	Dense accumulations of fibrous deposits within the cytoplasm of neurons, usually visualized in silver-stained brain sections. In AD, they are predominant in large pyramidal neurons of the neocortex and hippocampus.
Paired helical filaments (PHFs)	Electron-microscopic studies have shown that the NFTs of AD are made up of fine filaments that are twisted together to form regular paired helical structures.
Tau protein	The major protein constituent of the PHFs. It has recently been sequenced and is found to occur in 6 isoforms in the brain.
Senile (or neuritic) plaques	Extracellular tangles of neurites with a core of amyloid. Plaque deposits in the cortex and hippocampus are a second diagnostic neuropathologic feature of AD.
Amyloid	Amyloid is an extracellular deposit in many tissues that is defined by its particular optical properties when viewed under polarized light.
β/A 4 amyloid protein	The particular form of amyloid that is deposited in extracellular spaces and around blood vessels in AD. It has been sequenced and is found to consist of a 42 amino acid protein. It is thought to be an abnormal cleavage product of the precursor protein APP.
Amyloid precursor protein (APP)	Cloning of the β/A 4 protein has enabled the sequencing of the full APP precursor protein. There are 3 isoforms in the brain, 695, 751, and 770 amino acids long. APP is believed to be a membrane-bound protein, with the β/A 4 protein located close to its C-terminal end in the region thought to span the membrane. The function of APP in the intact CNS is at present unknown.

Introduction

As other chapters in this volume attest, the intracerebral grafting (ICG) of neural tissue is now well established as an effective strategy for anatomic reconstruction and functional repair in a variety of neural systems in the brain. Moreover, preliminary trials have commenced of the clinical applications of the ICG paradigm to a number of neurode-generative diseases, most notably parkinsonism (see chapter by Brundin and Lindvall, this volume). One of the fundamental conditions for the development of a rational ICG therapy is the identification of the target population(s) of cells central to the disease process, which one consequently seeks to replace. The failure as yet to identify the primary basis of the disease process in human dementia not only represents the biggest problem for developing an effective ICG strategy for the disease but restricts even the determination of the fundamental issue whether such a strategy might be feasible.

It would be impractical to attempt to repair in toto the variety of neurodegenerative events that have been considered to contribute to the mental deterioration in age- and disease-related dementia. Rather, the predominant approach in all research programs has been to seek to identify individual neuroanatomic or neurochemical systems that are either primary to the disease process or central to the functional deterioration. It would then be possible to attempt selective repair or replacement of the critical neural system(s) in order to inhibit the progression of the disease by blocking the process at an initial stage – e. g., to supply a deficient trophic factor or to inhibit amyloid deposition – before the more general secondary consequences have developed, or to restore aspects of impaired function that are of particular importance to the patient, e. g., memory.

Experimental ICG programs have been guided by a strategy of attempting restricted, focal repair of discrete identified systems critical for particular aspects of function. This means that the viability of the various strategies depends to a large degree on the validity of the hypotheses and animal models that underlie them. Thus, it is now well established that grafts of cholinergic neurons can alleviate some learning impairments associated with lesions of cholinergic systems in the rat forebrain (see below), but the applicability of the technique to human dementia depends in large part upon the validity in humans of the cholinergic hypothesis. The present chapter will describe a selection of the ICG approaches that have been adopted to correct cognitive deficits in experimental animal models of distinct components of the neuropathology of dementia and attempt to evaluate whether any point the way to a viable therapeutic strategy for the most widespread human neurodegenerative disease of our times.

Models of Cholinergic Deficiency

Cholinergic Hypothesis

Of the wide variety of neurochemical systems that degenerate in the aged brain, one of the most markedly and consistently affected is forebrain cholinergic function [1, 6, 8]. This was first noted as a decline in cortical and hippocampal choline acetyltransferase activity in the aged brain; there followed the observation that the basal forebrain neurons from which the cortical innervation arises also undergo aging- and dementia-related atrophy. Of particular interest in this context is the correlation between the decline in cortical cholinergic activity and that in mental test performance in demented patients, first established by Elaine Perry et al. [38] (Fig. 1). These several lines of research led to the cholinergic hypothesis of geriatric memory dysfunction, which proposes that deterioration in forebrain – particularly cortical – cholinergic systems underlies the cognitive deficits, es-

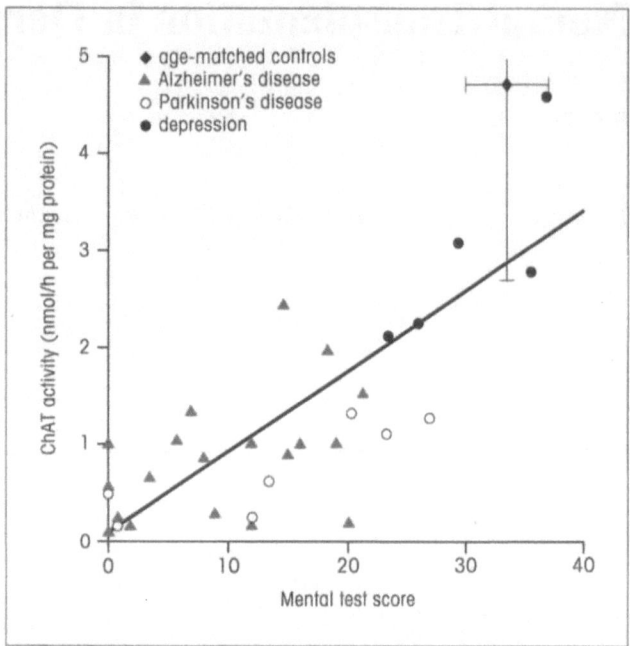

Fig. 1. *Correlation between the intellectual deficits in dementia and the decline in postmortem choline acetyltransferase (**ChAT**) activity in the temporal neocortex. The functional deficits were measured by means of a simple test of information and memory in patients with Alzheimer's disease, Parkinson's disease, or depression. The range of age-matched normal ChAT activity and test performance is shown by the **vertical** and **horizontal bars**. (After [37], with permission)*

pecially of learning and memory, that are associated with aging [1, 8]. This formulation of the problem has then provided the stimulus for an extensive search for cholinomimetic drugs that might provide a cholinergic replacement therapy for the cognitive deficits of aging and dementia; these drugs have largely been screened and tested for efficacy on animal models involving lesioning or pharmacologic blockade of the intrinsic forebrain systems.

Cholinergic Grafts in Rats and Monkeys with Lesions

In parallel with the pharmacologic studies, the effects of neural transplants rich in cholinergic neurons have been studied in rats with lesions of the basal forebrain cholinergic systems [10]. The techniques for transplantation of cholinergic neurons are straightforward (Fig. 2). The grafts require several months to grow and become well established within the host brain, which is necessary to allow time for extensive cholinergic-fiber reinnervation of the host targets.

Ventral forebrain grafts rich in cholinergic neurons can correct some of the learning deficits associated with lesions of forebrain cholinergic systems [10]. One of the first demonstrations of this phenomenon provides a good example of the general principles involved (Fig. 3). In this study [12], rats received lesions of the fimbria-fornix to deafferent the hippocampus of its main cholinergic (as well as adrener-

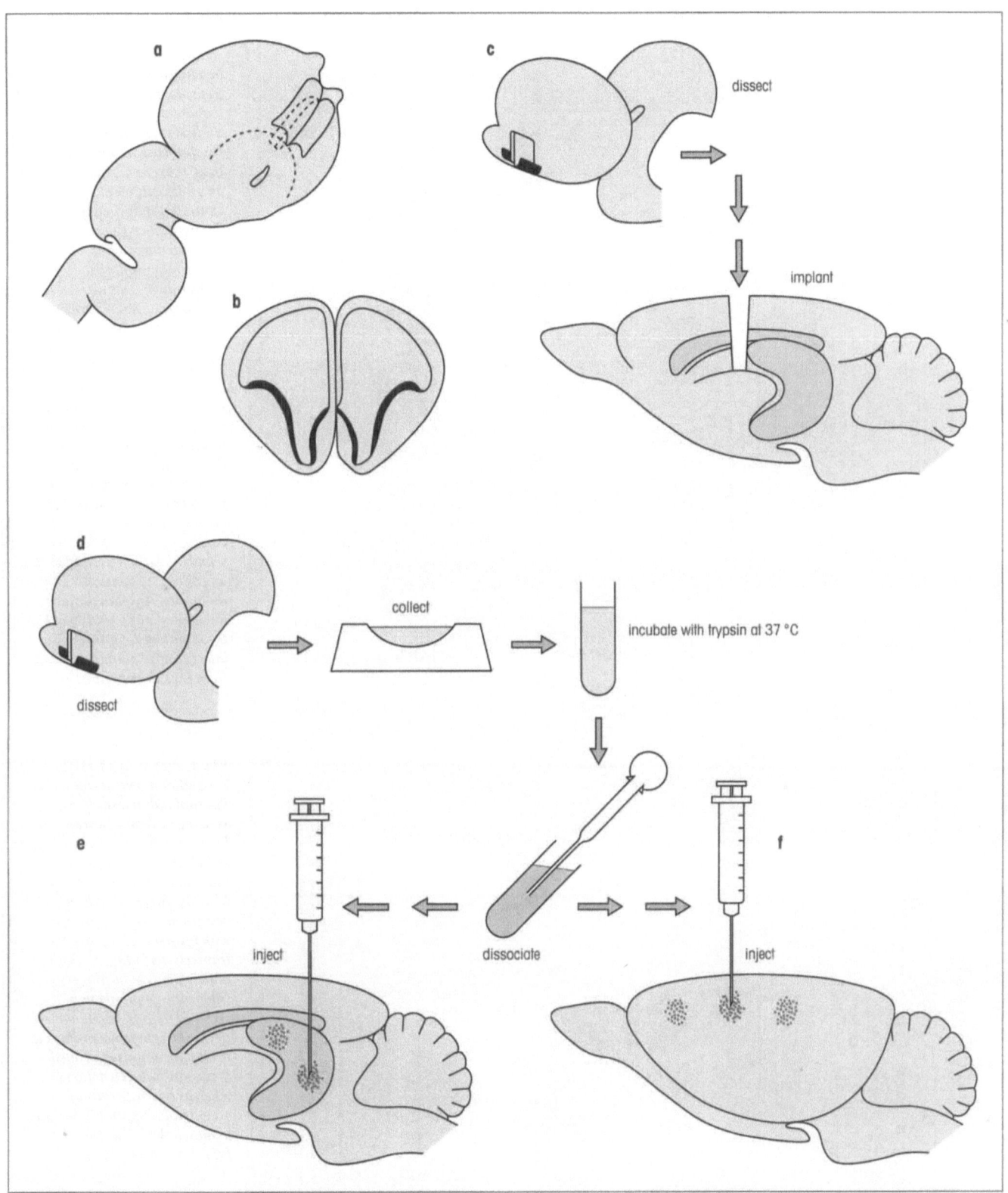

Fig. 2 a–f. *Techniques for the transplantation of acetylcholine(ACh-)-rich "septal" grafts from the basal forebrain region of embryos into the adult host cortex and hippocampus.* **a** *ACh-rich tissues are dissected from the ventral forebrain area of the embryonic brain, taken at 15–16 days of gestational age.* **b** *A coronal section through the rostral forebrain shows the ventromedial area containing the developing septal and diagonal band ACh neurons included in the dissection.* **c** *Solid grafts. The transplantations are made by implanting pieces of tissue into an appropriate cavity in the host brain. A cavity through the fimbria-fornix is shown, with the graft tissue positioned immediately next to the septal pole of the deafferented hippocampus.* **d** *Suspension grafts. The graft tissue from many embryos is pooled, digested in trypsin, washed, and mechanically dispersed to form a dissociated cell suspension that is injected stereotaxically in microliter portions into target sites in the adult host brain, such as the hippocampus (e) or the neocortex (f). (After [10], with permission)*

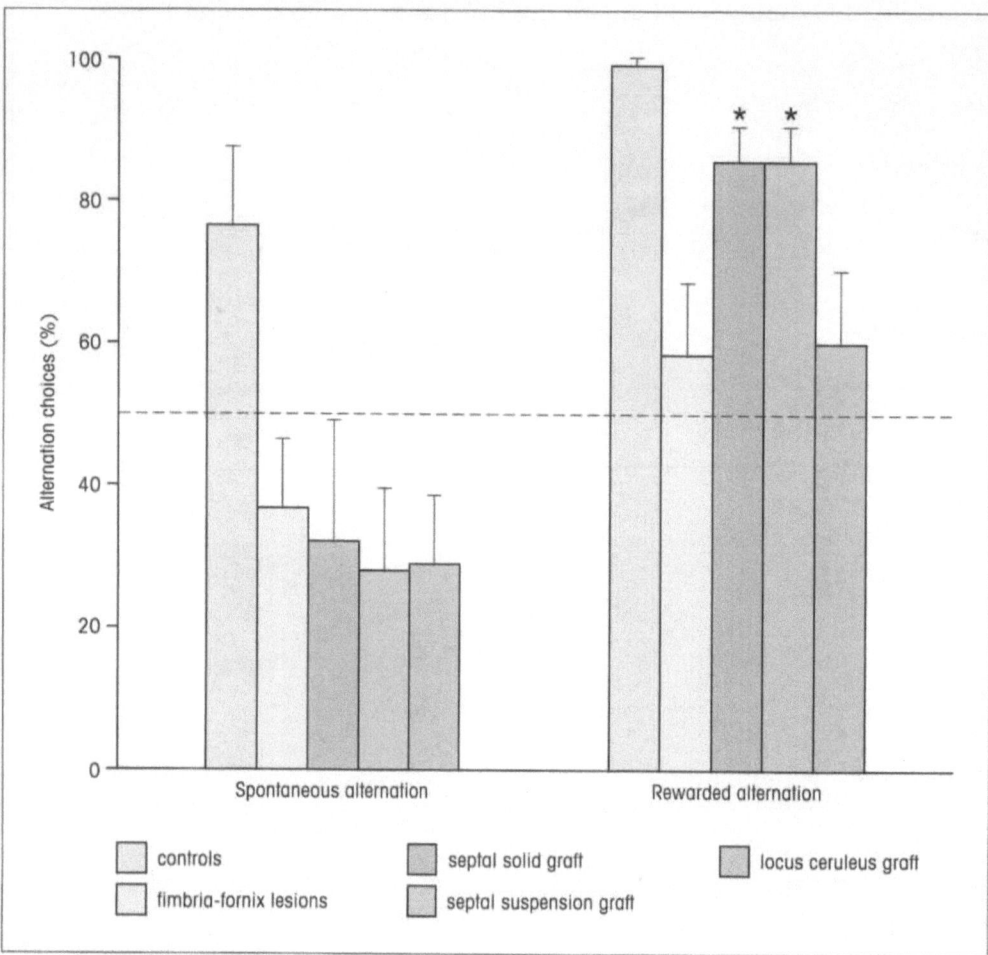

Fig. 3. *T-maze alternation performance in normal rats, rats with fimbria-fornix lesions, and lesioned rats after transplantation of alternative tissues into the hippocampus. In the first stage, the rats were tested for spontaneous alternation in the T-maze: whereas the controls alternated above chance level (**horizontal dashed line**), the lesions induced a pronounced side bias that was not affected by any type of graft. In the second stage, hungry rats were trained on rewarded alternation, i. e., given a food pellet each time they entered the arm opposite to that entered previously. Performance is shown on the final (eighth) week of training. The controls rapidly learned the task to a high level of performance, whereas the lesioned rats were unable to learn the task. Noradrenergic grafts of locus ceruleus tissue did not alleviate the deficit; by contrast, cholinergic grafts of septal cells (both as solid grafts and as cell suspensions) enabled the animals to learn the task (*), although they did not all achieve the same level of efficiency as intact control animals. (Data from [12], with permission)*

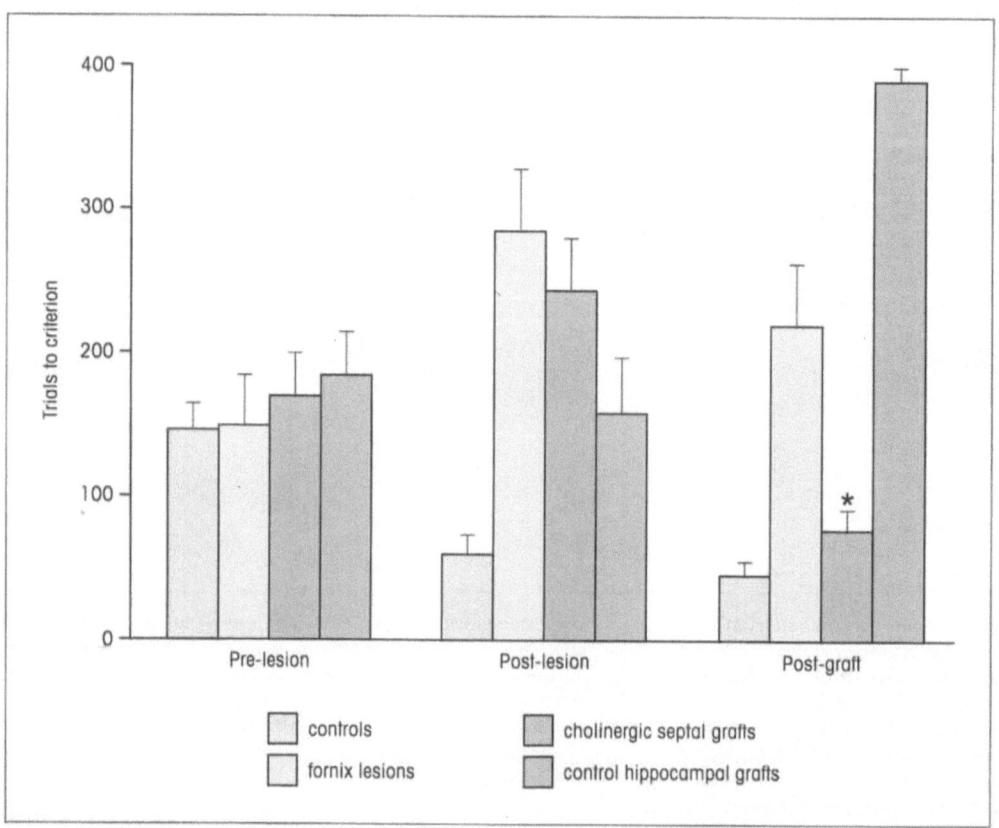

Fig. 4. *Learning of a series of conditional visuospatial discrimination tasks in the Wisconsin general test apparatus by marmosets with fornix lesions and cholinergic grafts. All marmosets were initially able to learn the first task. Whereas the control monkeys improved with further testing, fornix transections induced substantial impairments in the three subgroups of monkeys that received lesions. Implantation of cholinergic septal grafts into the hippocampus alleviated the lesion-induced deficit (*), whereas control grafts of acetylcholine-poor hippocampal tissue was without effect. (After [43], with permission)*

gic and serotoninergic) inputs, followed by grafts of either embryonic ventral forebrain (rich in cholinergic neurons) or embryonic locus ceruleus (rich in noradrenergic neurons). The lesions produced a profound deficit both in spontaneous exploratory behavior (measured in terms of spontaneous alternation in a T-maze) and in the animals' abilities to learn a spatial alternation task in the T-maze. Whereas noradrenergic grafts had no effect whatsoever on the animals' maze-learning deficit, the cholinergic grafts provided a substantial and significant improvement.

Several features of this experiment suggest that the effects are relatively specific. (1) The critical feature for functional recovery was the grafts' containing cholinergic cells rather than whether the grafts were made by the solid or the cell-suspension method. (2) A cholinergic reinnervation of the denervated hippocampus was sufficient to restore a limited degree of function, even though the full septohippocampal circuitry was not reconstructed. (3) Cholinergic reinnervation of the host hippocampus appeared to be a necessary but not a sufficient condition for functional repair, since in individual cases a return of acetylcholinesterase staining was not attended by functional recovery. (4) Although the effective grafts improved performance significantly, even the best grafted animals still learned the task substantially slower than control animals.

Reconstruction of the cholinergic inputs alone thus appears to be insufficient to restore normal performance, and further reconstruction may be necessary for full functional recovery, either by better integration of the grafted neurons or by restitution of some other neural system(s) disrupted by the lesions, e. g., noradrenergic or serotoninergic afferents to the hippocampus or efferent projections coursing via the fimbria-fornix to subcortical sites. Subsequent experiments have thrown further light on these issues.

First, the ability of cholinergic grafts in the hippocampus to correct deficits associated with fimbria-fornix or septal lesions has been confirmed in a wide variety of learning paradigms, including T-mazes, radial mazes, water mazes, and an operant timing task [9, 10, 13]. In addition, similar principles have been found to apply also in the neocortex, the other major projection target of the cholinergic forebrain system; thus, cholinergic grafts implanted into the neocortex have been found to correct deficits induced by lesions of the basal forebrain in passive avoidance, water maze, T-maze, and attentional operant tasks [9, 10].

Second, several of these studies have used additional pharmacologic manipulations to show that the graft-derived recovery is attributable to a specific cholinergic mechanism. Thus, Nilsson et al. have demonstrated that the recovery in the Morris water maze induced by septal grafts could be blocked by the muscarinic antagonist atropine, whereas this drug had no effect on the rats with lesions alone [32]. In a comprehensive series of studies, Hodges et al. have used a complex radial maze task that enabled them to identify lesion and graft effects separately on both working and reference memory components of maze learning based on the use of both spatial and nonspatial cues [24, 25]. Grafts implanted into the hippocampus produced substantial amelioration of both

spatial and cue-based reference memory and complete recovery of both spatial and cue-based working memory [24]. Both the muscarinic agonist arecoline and the nicotinic agonist nicotine enhanced the performance of the lesioned rats, but had no effect (arecoline) on, or actually impaired (nicotine), the already efficient performance of control rats or rats with lesions plus cortical or hippocampal grafts. By contrast, scopolamine and mecamylamine, antagonists at the two major classes of cholinergic receptors, were found to disrupt the performance of the control and grafted rats, while having less effect on the rats receiving lesions alone [25].

Third, these observations have recently been extended from rodents to a small New World primate, the common marmoset, in an elegant series of studies by Ridley and Baker [43]. They have used a series of tasks, involving learning and reversal of simple and complex visual and visuospatial discriminations, to characterize the deficits that result from disruptions in the septohippocampal system. They have found not only that conditional visuospatial discriminations appear to be particularly sensitive to fornix transection, but also that grafts of cholinergic tissue from marmoset fetuses (but not control grafts of cholinergic-poor tissue) can, when implanted into the hippocampus of lesioned monkeys, alleviate these deficits (Fig. 4).

Fourth, several recent studies suggest that the age of the graft donor may be critical for the functional effect. Thus, whereas grafts derived from embryos at all ages from E 13 to E 17 appear to give rise to good cholinergic reinnervation of the hippocampus, only host animals bearing grafts from the younger E 13 and E 14 donors appear to show satisfactory functional recovery in both radial-maze und operant tasks [4, 13]. This has been taken to support the hypothesis that some neuronal connections other than just cholinergic must underlie the functional recovery.

Fifth, a first clue to which additional systems are possibly involved comes from the demonstration that cografts of serotoninergic raphe tissue can substantially augment the benefit derived from cholinergic grafts, even though raphe grafts on their own generally exert no significant effect [33, 42]. This supports Vanderwolf's recent hypothesis that the serotoninergic systems modulate cholinergic function in the hippocampus [52] and is compatible with his observations that blocking both systems together induces far greater deficits than disturbing either system alone.

Cholinergic Grafts in Aging Animals

The fact that old rats and monkeys show deficits on many tests of learning and memory similar to those seen in animals with septohippocampal lesions or given anticholinergic drugs has been taken both to give credence to the cholinergic hypothesis of geriatric cognitive deficits and to provide a rationale for testing potential cholinergic replacement strategies in old rats. Cholinomimetic drugs have provided significant effects in a few model systems [1], but generally the efficacy of both direct receptor agonists and anticholinesterase inhibitors in aged animals has been disap-

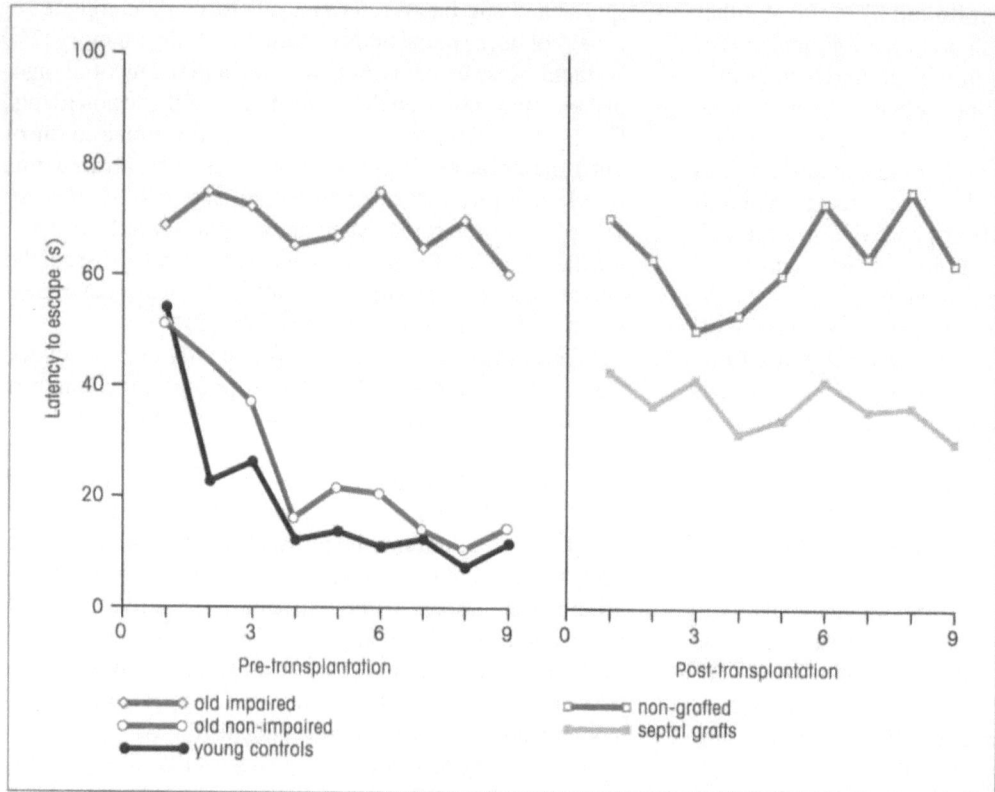

Fig. 5. *Recovery of spatial navigation in the Morris water maze task in successive blocks of four trials before and after transplantation of septal tissue into the hippocampus of impaired old rats. In this task, the animals must learn to escape from a large swimming pool full of water by finding an escape platform located in a constant spatial position in every trial. Whereas young animals learn to swim directly to the platform within 15–20 trials, 30%–40% of 20-month-old rats cannot learn the task (**open diamonds, left panel**). A subset of the old impaired animals received septal grafts and manifested marked improvements in performance when tested again 3 months later (**filled squares, right panel**), whereas the rats without transplants (**open squares, right panel**) did not improve, despite further training. (After [20], with permission)*

pointing. By contrast, several studies have revealed quite substantial benefits, albeit on selected tasks, of cholinergic-rich neural grafts in aged animals [9, 10].

In the first study of the functional effects of ICG on age-related learning deficits, Gage et al. [20] screened a large group of old rats in the Morris water-maze task and selected 17 that manifested learning impairments greater than two standard deviations outside the range of performance of young rats tested in parallel. The aged rats were subdivided, one group receiving cholinergic septal suspension grafts implanted into the hippocampus, exactly as described above for lesioned rats (see Fig. 2E). Three months were allowed for the grafts to grow and integrate with the host brain before the rats were retested in the water-maze task (Fig. 5). The old rats with grafts showed substantial improvement over their previous levels of impairment, whereas those without grafts showed no improvement whatsoever. Even within the grafted group, two of the ten rats remained as impaired as the old rats without grafts, which was accounted for in the subsequent histologic examination by a failure of the grafts to thrive in just these two cases [20]. The other eight grafted rats recovered to a level that was not significantly different from that of either the young rats or the old but unimpaired rats.

Subsequently, ICG studies in aged rats have been extended to consider issues similar to those already addressed in lesioned animals (see the preceding section). First, the recovery in the water maze induced by cholinergic septal grafts implanted into the hippocampus of aged rats has been shown to be by an atropine-dependent (i.e., presumably cholinergic) mechanism [18]. Second, the benefits of such grafts have been shown to extend to other tasks, including operant delayed matching to sample [14]. Third, similar principles are found to apply with cholinergic grafts implanted in the neocortex as with grafts in the hippocampus of aged rats [14]. Fourth, recovery on other types of task or classes of behavioral impairment can be obtained after the implantation of other types of tissue into the hippocampus or other target areas in aged rats; thus, hippocampal implantation of noradrenergic grafts can alleviate aged rats' deficits in the acquisition and retention of a passive avoidance task [5], and intrastriatal implantation of dopaminergic nigral grafts can correct deficits in motor coordination and balance [19]. Interestingly, the last-mentioned study was conducted in parallel with the one described above of the effects of septal grafts on the water-maze performance of aged rats, and the patterns of recovery (in motor versus spatial learning tasks) were quite specific to the transmitter produced by the graft and the site of implantation [19, 20].

Models of Trophic Factor Deficiency

Role of NGF in Trophic Support

A tangential development of the cholinergic hypothesis has been the hypothesis that the cholinergic deficit in Alzheimer's disease is due to a deficiency in specific trophic factors. This hypothesis has derived from the discovery that basal forebrain cholinergic neurons are dependent upon target-derived nerve growth factor (NGF) for trophic support. The demonstration that these same cholinergic neurons degenerate in Alzheimer's disease prompted Hefti [23] to suggest the insufficient availability of NGF. Although there have been difficulties in demonstrating any consistent reduction of NGF levels, NGF receptors, or NGF expression in the cortex or hippocampus of the postmortem Alzheimer brain, Fischer et al. [17] have found that chronic NGF administration can block the development of both the atrophy of septal cholinergic neurons and the impairments in retention of spatial navigation learning between blocks of test sessions in aged rats.

Although this suggests that NGF replacement might be a useful therapeutic strategy for Alzheimer's disease, there is a practical difficulty: in order to be effective, NGF must be administered intracerebrally and chronically. The problem is not insurmountable, as evidenced by the introduction of the intracerebral delivery of NGF to promote the viability of adrenal grafts in parkinsonian patients [35]. Alternatively, cell tranplants might provide a more effective system for the delivery of NGF than chronic intracerebral infusions.

Transplants as NGF Delivery Systems

Various tissues naturally rich in NGF have been used both to promote the viability of NGF-dependent cells after ICG and to inhibit the degeneration of cholinergic neurons after axotomy [9]. For instance, implants of mouse submaxillary gland have been shown to increase the survival of septal and diagonal band neurons after fimbria-fornix transection [48]. However, even surviving neurons are unable to regrow across the lesion cavity to reinnervate their hippocampal targets, unless a bridge of suitable tissue is provided as a substrate [29]. Messersmith et al. [31] made sciatic nerve implants into fimbria-fornix cavities in an attempt to combine the secretory and the supporting function; indeed, this resulted in an increased concentration of NGF in the host septum and provided a substrate for substantial cholinergic fiber growth. However, these studies have not shown that the enhanced survival of septal cholinergic cells is any greater when they reconnect with their targets than when NGF is supplied diffusely, nor have they shown that the extent of fiber outgrowth across the bridge into the hippocampus is any greater than when other suitable but less NGF-rich substrates for growth are used.

Genetically modified cells may constitute an alternative source for achieving the sustained delivery of physiologic levels of NGF [21] (see the chapter by Gage and Fisher, this volume). Considerable preliminary success has been achieved in the transfection of fibroblasts and maintained cell lines with a variety of reporter genes (such as that for β-galactosidase) and neuroactive genes (including the NGF gene). Such cells can have biologic activity after transplantation: for instance, intraventricular implants of NGF-secreting cells can rescue septal cholinergic neurons from the retrograde death induced by axotomy [22, 42] (Fig. 6), although the functional efficacy of such grafts is still largely unknown.

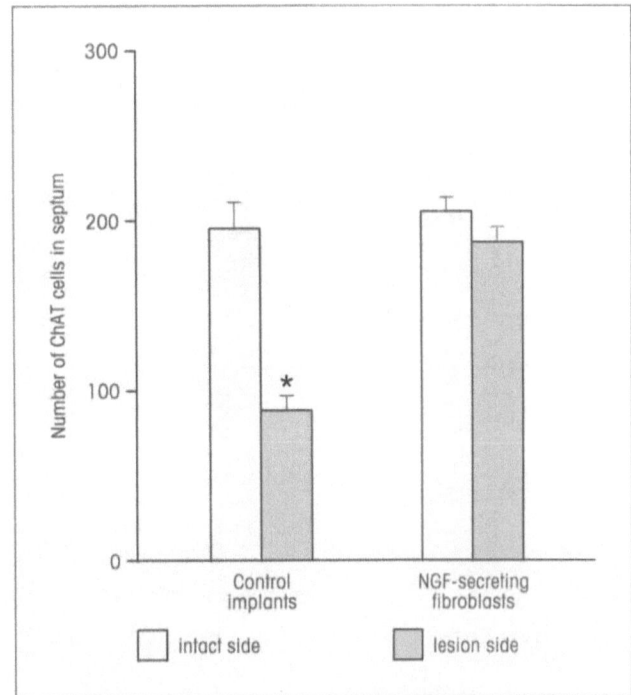

Fig. 6. *Intraventricular implants of NGF-secreting fibroblasts promote the survival of axotomized septal cholinergic neurons. All animals received a unilateral fimbria-fornix lesion to transect the septohippocampal axons on one side. In animals with NGF-secreting grafts, the number of cells surviving on the side of the lesion was almost equal to that on the intact side. (After [44], with permission)*

Critical Neuropathology of Alzheimer's Disease

The studies mentioned in the preceding sections have all been based on the ICG of identified populations of subcortical neurons – predominantly cholinergic, but also dopaminergic, noradrenergic, and serotoninergic – in neurotransmitter-specific models of dementia. The validity of this approach, however, has been the subject of an increasing number of challenges. There is no dispute about the fact that these systems do undergo various degrees of decline in the aging or demented brain. Nor is there any dispute about the fact that experimental disturbance of these individual systems in young animals – whether by drugs, toxins, or lesions – can disrupt cognitive functions measured by their performance in mazes and other learning or memory tasks. Rather, it appears increasingly likely that the changes in subcortical neuronal systems are secondary to the fundamental degenerative process in dementia. Consequently, whereas it may be possible to induce functional recovery with a pharmacologically specific, e.g., cholinomimetic, treatment when experimental damage is restricted to a disturbance of the cholinergic regulation of the cortex or hippocampus, it is quite unlikely that such a treatment will have any beneficial effect when the cholinergic loss in accompanied by the widespread degeneration of the cortical or hippocampal targets that occurs in various dementing diseases, whichever component of the degeneration turns out to be primary.

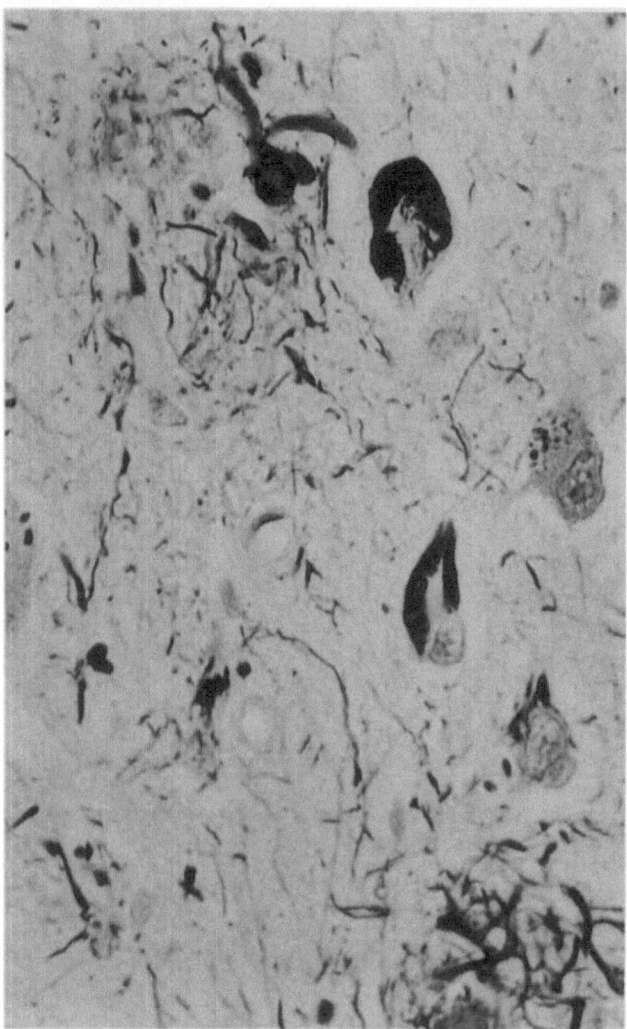

Fig. 7. Senile plaques and neurofibrillary tangles: the classical hall-marks of cortical and hippocampal degeneration in Alzheimer's disease. Palmgren silver stain. (Courtesy of Dr. D. M. A. Mann, University of Manchester, UK)

Cortical and Subcortical Cell Loss

Prior to the relatively recent interest in identified neuro-chemical systems in the forebrain, dementia was primarily associated with neuropathologic changes in the neocortex. This can include widespread cell loss, atrophy of the cortical mantle, and enlargement of the ventricles, as well as the classical senile plaques and neurofibrillary tangles of Alzheimer's disease (Fig. 7) and the multiple foci of perivascular degeneration in multiinfarct dementia [30, 51]. The view that the symptomatology of dementia, involving a global impairment of intellect, reason, and personality, as well as pronounced deficits in memory and learning, may best be considered "the result of a more or less extensive destruction or disorganization of the cerebral cortex" [50] is still not misplaced [30, 36]. The subcortical cell loss, e. g., in cholinergic systems, may then be most appropriately viewed as a secondary retrograde response to cortical degeneration [36].

ICG strategies have been used both to study this retrograde response and to attempt structural repair of the damaged neocortex. Thus, Sofroniew et al. have used excitotoxins to lesion cortical neurons without inducing direct destruction of the afferent cholinergic terminals [45]. Such lesions result in retrograde atrophy of cholinergic neurons in the basal forebrain. However, the survival of these cholinergic cells can be promoted by target replacement, achieved by implanting embryonic neocortical tissue into the denervated neocortex [46]. Although the cortical grafts were seen to be reinnervated by host cholinergic axons, the grafted cells did not establish long-distance efferent connections with the host brain, and they were consequently without effect on the functional deficits induced by the cortical lesions in the host animals [47].

Amyloid, Plaques, and Tangles in Dementia

Over the past 5–7 years, there has been a dramatic resurgence in research on Alzheimer's disease with the identification of the amino acid structure of the $\beta/A4$ amyloid protein, which constitutes the core of the senile plaque, and of the amyloid precursor protein (APP), from which it is cleaved [28]. In parallel, the contribution of tau protein and other neurofilament proteins to the neurofibrillary tangles is now well described [53], although the precise structural and neurochemical composition of the neurofilaments is still not clear. These developments are leading to fundamental new insights into the ways in which abnormal expression, processing, and cleavage of normal proteins can induce a cascade of events that end up in the characteristic neuronal degeneration of Alzheimer's disease.

Graft Models of the Cellular Pathology of Alzheimer's Disease

In the light of these developments in understanding the neuropathologic changes of Alzheimer's disease and other dementias, several recent studies have employed neural tranplants in the search for better models of the underlying neurodegenerative processes. To date, these models are restricted to the demonstration and analysis of the pathologic cellular changes; they have not yet been evaluated within the context of functional analysis or repair.

Cellular Pathology in Aging Grafts

One approach has been to employ neural transplantation strategies to investigate long-term cellular aging processes in isolated tissues. For example, Olson, Eriksdotter-Nilsson et al. have followed the survival and anatomic development of cerebellar and hippocampal tissues over 22–23 months after transplantation in the anterior chamber of the eye. In the aged grafts, marked differences in neuronal organization, an increased gliosis, and a marked accumulation of autofluorescent lipofuscin granules were seen to develop [15, 16], all of which are characteristic features of the normal aging process in the brain.

A second approach has been to focus on morphological changes in the neurons or glia of aging grafts. One intriguing observation has been the demonstration of Hirano bodies and immunoreactivity with neurofilament antibodies – both of which are characteristic of tangle-bearing cortical and hippocampal neurons in Alzheimer's disease – in CNS grafts isolated for longer than 6 months in a peripheral transplantation site [7]. However, other markers of senile plaques or neurofibrillary tangles, such as staining with Congo red, thioflavin-S or antibodies against paired helical filaments, were not observed in these grafts. Nevertheless, these observations provided a clear demonstration of the accumulation of individual features of the human neuropathology in isolated grafts and offer model systems in which their development might be studied experimentally [7].

Trisomy 16 Transplant Model

A novel approach to the induction of Alzheimer-like pathologic changes in grafts has recently been described; it is based on the established association between Down syndrome, Alzheimer's disease, and human chromosome 21 [34, 40]. Since many genes and markers on human chromosome 21 map to chromosome 16 in the mouse, it was suggested that trisomy 16 in mice might provide an animal model not only of human Down syndrome but also of the neuropathologic features of Alzheimer's disease. It had been difficult to address this issue, since trisomy 16 fetuses do not survive beyond term. However, neural transplantation of embryonic trisomy 16 tissue into normal host mice has recently been employed to study the long-term development of proteins encoded by chromosome 16 genes [26] and of characteristic neuropathologic features of Alzheimer's disease [41].

In the studies by Richards et al. [40, 41], neocortex and hippocampus were transplanted from trisomy 16 embryos or littermate control embryos into the frontal and retrosplenial cortex, respectively, of normal young adult host mice. A variety of neuropathologic changes characteristic of Alzheimer's disease were identified immunocytochemically in the trisomic grafts after 4 months survival (Table 1). In particular, a granular pattern of intracellular amyloid and tau immunoreactivity was observed in neurons both from the grafts and in Alzheimer brain (Fig. 8). No similar immunoreactivity was seen either in control grafts from normal littermates or in the trisomic embryos.

Similar observations have recently been reported by Epstein et al. in long-term (4–6 months) reaggregate trisomy 16 cultures [2], but other graft studies have either failed to reproduce the abnormal amyloid deposition [49] or have reported a more rapid time course of pathologic expression in the trisomy 16 grafts [27]. Thus, further analysis is required to identify more precisely the subpopulation of

Table 1. *Patterns of neuropathologic staining in trisomy 16 grafts (from data in [40] and [41])*

Antibody or stain	Host brain	Control graft	Trisomy 16 graft
Thioflavin-S	–	–	Intracellular
Palmgren silver	Fibers	Fibers	Fibers and intracellular
Amyloid precursor protein	–	–	Intracellular and extracellular
β/A4 amyloid protein	–	–	Intracellular
α_1-Antichymotrypsin	–	–	Intracellular and extracellular
Paired helical filaments	–	–	Intracellular
Tau protein (6.423)	–	–	Intracellular
Glial fibrillary acidic protein	Astrocytes	Cell bodies	Astrocyte processes
Ubiquitin	Processes	Processes	Processes and occasional cell bodies

cells in which the characteristic pathologic changes develop and to resolve the observations of abnormal immunocytochemical staining at the ultrastructural level in order to identify the abnormal elements within the cells of trisomy 16 grafts. Nevertheless, this paradigm provides perhaps the first viable animal model not only for monitoring the development of the cellular changes involved in the human disease, but also for assessing alternative therapeutic strategies aimed at inhibiting or reversing the pathogenetic process.

Future Prospects for Better Functional Animal Models

As noted above, transplantation models have so far been restricted to the development and analysis of the neuropathologic cellular changes of Alzheimer's disease in experimental animals and have not yet progressed to studies of the potential of grafts for functional repair. There are now several techniques for mimicking individual neuropathologic features of dementia [11]. For example, the intracerebral inoculation of mice with certain strains of the scrapie virus can induce extensive spongiform encephalopathy and amyloid plaque formation, and deficits in passive avoidance can be detected even before the appearance of overt pathologic changes. Alternatively, intracerebral injection of high concentrations of aluminum salts has been seen to induce the formation of widespread neurofibrillary degeneration in rabbits, cats, and rats, and is associated with impairments in learning tasks as well as the pronounced ataxia and motor impairments that lead to rapid death in this model. However, neither the scrapie nor the aluminum model reproduces the actual pathologic elements involved in the human disease, with respect either to the distribution of neuropathologic changes or to the detailed molecular structure of the associated neurofibrillary deposits [11]. A better approach may be the recent development of strains of transgenic mice

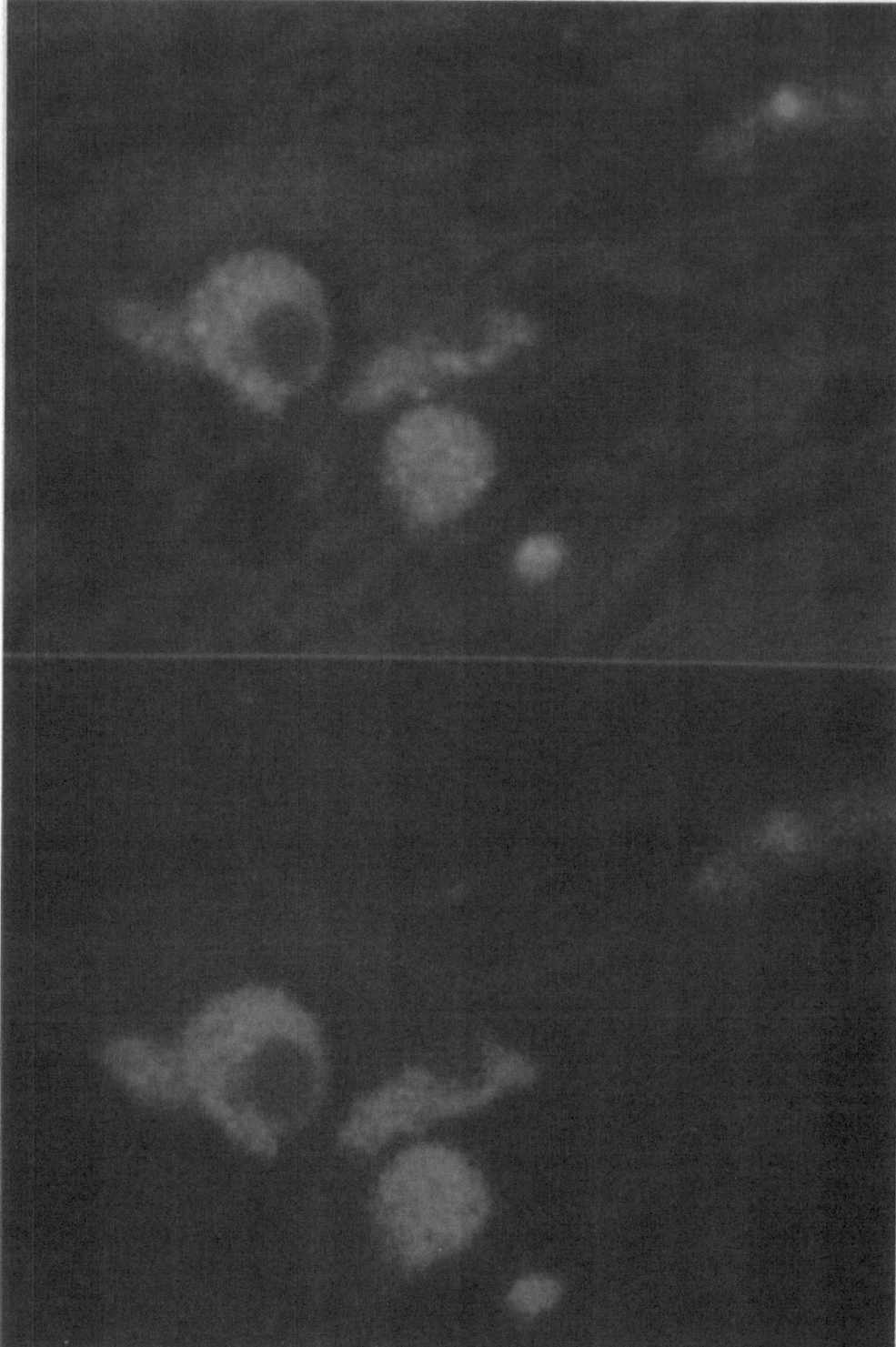

Fig. 8 a, b. *Trisomy 16 grafts manifest cellular pathology akin to that in Alzheimer's disease.* **a** *Trisomy 16 neurons stained with an antibody against the β/A 4 protein.* **b** *The same neurons visualized with the Tau 6.423 monoclonal antibody. Note the granular pattern of cytoplasmic labeling and the colocalization of the two epitopes within the same cells. (From [41], with permission)*

that overexpress particular isoforms of the amyloid precursor protein gene [39], and at least one such strain manifests mild but significant deficits in learning the Morris water maze spatial navigation task [54]. Although these various approaches may provide functional models of particular aspects of the cellular neuropathology that underlies human dementia, unfortunately none have yet been used to evaluate possibilities of repair by ICG.

Clinical Prospects in Dementia

To summarize the studies in experimental animals, neural transplants have been demonstrated to have at least a limited capacity to reconstruct identified neurotransmitter systems in the brain and to provide functional recovery on relevant behavioral tests of cognitive function. This applies in particular to neuronal systems that are highly branched and diffuse in their distribution and probably function to provide a regulation of their target structures (such as the cholinergic, serotoninergic, or dopaminergic neurons of the isodendritic core), rather than to systems involved in the precise point-to-point relay of information between processing centers of the brain.

Although such observations have occasionally been taken to be relevant to human dementia, in particular within the context of the cholinergic hypothesis, the present review considers this optimism to be misplaced, except perhaps in particular, circumscribed circumstances. Thus, the cholinergic deficit may indeed be central to some of the cognitive deficits in natural aging. It may also be relevant to certain dementias of subcortical origin, in particular in Parkinson's disease, in which cell loss and Lewy body degeneration occur in the basal nucleus of Meynert as well as in the substantia nigra [3] in the absence of any overt cortical or hippocampal degeneration. However, it is unlikely that ICG would be warranted in these conditions – either because the disorder is not sufficiently debilitating (e. g., the increasing forgetfulness associated with normal aging) or because the cognitive disorder is a consideration secondary to more profound problems (such as the motor disorder of advanced parkinsonism).

By contrast, the available data suggest that the predominant dementing diseases of the Alzheimer and multiinfarct types involve extensive degeneration and cell loss in the neocortex and the allocortex that cannot be attributed to a primary loss of circumscribed populations of subcortical regulatory systems. It is not possible to reconstruct such widespread target degeneration by replacing individual regulatory inputs. To date, the experimental repair of complex cortical circuits by ICG in adult animals has proved to have only limited success, and in those cases in which benefit has been positively demonstrated it is almost certainly due to relatively nonspecific neurotrophic processes rather than to reconstruction of the damaged circuitry by the grafts. It should be noted that extensive reconstruction in complex neural circuits is not ruled out in principle, as evidenced by the degree of recovery that can be achieved by ICG in neostriatal systems. Rather, the conditions for similar patterns of repair of the neocortex have not yet been identified.

It is likely that our rapidly expanding understanding of the molecular and genetic events that give rise to the cellular degeneration and abnormal amyloid and neurofibrillary deposits in Alzheimer's disease will lead to novel strategies for inhibiting the pathologic process of dementia and repairing damaged cortical structures. Indeed, ICG techniques are contributing to the development of new pathogenetic models, and it is plausible that they will also come to play a role in the treatment of dementing diseases. However, such advances are at present entirely speculative and will be possible only when the principal neuronal elements and primary pathologic processes involved in Alzheimer's disease and other dementias are finally identified and understood.

Acknowledgements. I thank Dr. David Mann for providing the color photomicrograph reproduced in Fig. 7 and Drs. E. H. Perry, F. H. Gage, S.-J. Richards, and E. K. Rosenberg for permission to reproduce figures or data from their publications. Our own studies have been supported by grants from the Mental Health Foundation, the Medical Research Council, and Sandoz Pharmaceuticals.

References

1. Bartus RT, Dean RL, Beer B, Lippa AS (1982) The cholinergic hypothesis of geriatric memory dysfunction. Science 217: 408–417
2. Bredesen DE, Kane DJ, Holtzman DM, Epstein CJ (1991) Re-aggregating cultures of trisomy 16 brain. Soc Neurosci Abstr 17: 1064
3. Candy JM, Perry RH, Perry EK, Irving D, Blessed G, Fairbairn AF, Tomlinson BE (1983) Pathological changes in the nucleus of Meynert in Alzheimer's and Parkinson's diseases. J Neurol Sci 54: 277–289
4. Cassel JC, Kelche C, Peterson GM, Ballough GP, Goepp I, Will B (1991) Graft-induced behavioral recovery from subcallosal septo-hippocampal damage in rats depends on maturity stage of donor tissue. Neuroscience 45: 571–586
5. Collier TJ, Gash DM, Sladek JR (1988) Transplantation of norepinephrine neurons into aged rats improves performance of a learned task. Brain Res 448: 77–87
6. Coyle JT, Price DL, DeLong MR (1983) Alzheimer's disease: a disorder of cortical cholinergic innervation. Science 219: 1184–1190
7. Doering LC, Aguayo AJ (1987) Hirano bodies and other cytoskeletal abnormalities in fetal rat CNS grafts isolated for long periods in peripheral nerve. Brain Res 401: 178–184
8. Drachman DA, Sahakian BJ (1980) Memory, aging and pharmacosystems. In: Stein D (ed) The psychobiology of aging: problems and perspectives. Elsevier/North Holland, Amsterdam, pp 347–368
9. Dunnett SB (1990) Neural transplantation in animal models of dementia. Eur J Neurosci 2: 567–587
10. Dunnett SB (1991) Cholinergic grafts, ageing and memory in rats. Trends Neurosci 14: 371–376
11. Dunnett SB, Barth TM (1991) Animal models of Alzheimer's disease and dementia. In: Willner P (ed) Behavioural models in psychopharmacology. Cambridge University Press, London, pp 359–418
12. Dunnett SB, Low WC, Iversen SD, Stenevi U, Björklund A (1982) Septal transplants restore maze learning in rats with fornix-fimbria lesions. Brain Res 251: 335–348
13. Dunnett SB, Martel FL, Rogers DC, Finger S (1989) Factors affecting septal graft amelioration of differential reinforcement of low rates (DRL) and activity deficits after fimbria-fornix lesions. Restor Neurol Neurosci 1: 83–92
14. Dunnett SB, Badman F, Rogers DC, Evenden JL, Iversen SD (1989) Cholinergic grafts in the neocortex or hippocampus of aged rats: reduction of delay-dependent deficits in the delayed non-matching to position task. Exp Neurol 102: 57–64
15. Eriksdotter-Nilsson M, Gerhardt G, Seiger Å, Hoffer B, Granholm A-C (1989) Multiple changes in noradrenergic mechanisms in the coeruleo-hippocampal pathway during aging. Structural and functional correlates in intraocular double grafts. Neurobiol Aging 10: 117–124
16. Eriksdotter-Nilsson M, Gerhardt G, Seiger Å, Olson L, Hoffer B, Granholm A-C (1989) Age-related alterations in noradrenergic input to the hippocampal formation: structural and functional studies in intraocular transplants. Brain Res 478: 269–280
17. Fischer W, Wictorin K, Björklund A, Williams LR, Varon S, Gage FH (1987) Amelioration of cholinergic neuron atrophy and spatial memory impairment in aged rats by nerve growth factor. Nature 329: 65–68

18. Gage FH, Björklund A (1986) Cholinergic septal grafts into the hippocampal formation improve spatial learning and memory in aged rats by an atropine-sensitive mechanism. J Neurosci 6: 2837–2847

19. Gage FH, Dunnett SB, Stenevi U, Björklund A (1983) Aged rats: recovery of motor impairment by intrastriatal nigral grafts. Science 221: 966–969

20. Gage FH, Björklund A, Stenevi U, Dunnett SB, Kelly PAT (1984) Intrahippocampal septal grafts ameliorate learning deficits in aged rats. Science 225: 533–536

21. Gage FH, Wolff JA, Rosenberg MB, Xu L, Yee J-K, Shults C, Friedmann T (1987) Grafting genetically modified cells to the brain: possibilities for the future. Neuroscience 23: 795–807

22. Gage FH, Fisher LJ, Jinnah JHA, Rosenberg MB, Tuszynski M, Friedmann T (1990) Grafting genetically modified cells to the brain: conceptual and technical issues. Prog Brain Res 82: 1–10

23. Hefti F, Weiner WJ (1986) Nerve growth factor and Alzheimer's disease. Ann Neurol 20: 275–281

24. Hodges H, Allen Y, Kershaw T, Lantos PL, Gray JA, Sinden J (1991) Effects of cholinergic-rich neural grafts on radial maze performance of rats after excitotoxic lesions of the forebrain cholinergic projection system: I. Amelioration of cognitive deficits by transplants into cortex and hippocampus but not into basal forebrain. Neuroscience 45: 587–607

25. Hodges H, Allen Y, Kershaw T, Lantos PL, Gray JA, Sinden J (1991) Effects of cholinergic-rich neural grafts on radial maze performance of rats after excitotoxic lesions of the forebrain cholinergic projection system: II. Cholinergic drugs as probes to investigate lesion-induced deficits and transplant-induced functional recovery. Neuroscience 45: 609–623

26. Höhmann CF, Capone G, Oster-Granite M-L, Coyle JT (1990) Transplantation of brain tissue from murine trisomy 16 into euploid hosts: effects of gene imbalance on brain development. Prog Brain Res 82: 203–214

27. Höhmann CF, Capone GT, Diggs AM, Coyle JT (1991) Expression of amyloid in cortical transplants of trisomy 16 mouse. Soc Neurosci Abstr 17: 51

28. Kang J, Lemaire HG, Unterbeck A, Salbaum M, Masters CL, Grzeschik KH, Multhaup G Beyreuther K, Muller-Hill B (1987) The precursor of Alzheimer's disease amyloid protein resembles a cell-surface receptor. Nature 325: 733–736

29. Kromer LF, Björklund A, Stenevi U (1981) Regeneration of the septohippocampal pathways in adult rats is promoted by utilizing embryonic hippocampal implants as bridges. Brain Res 210: 173–200

30. Mann DMA (1988) Neuropathological and neurochemical aspects of Alzheimer's disease. In: Iversen LL, Iversen SD, Snyder SH (eds) Handbook of psychopharmacology, vol 20. Plenum, New York, pp 1–67

31. Messersmith DJ, Fabrazzo M, Mocchetti I, Kromer LF (1991) Effects of sciatic nerve transplants after fimbria-fornix lesion: examination of the role of nerve growth factor. Brain Res 557: 293–297

32. Nilsson OG, Shapiro ML, Olton DS, Gage FH, Björklund A (1987) Spatial learning and memory following fimbria-fornix transection and grafting of fetal septal neurons to the hippocampus. Exp Brain Res 67: 195–215

33. Nilsson OG, Brundin P, Björklund A (1990) Amelioration of spatial memory impairment by intrahippocampal grafts of mixed septal and raphe tissue in rats with combined cholinergic and serotonergic denervation of the forebrain. Brain Res 515: 193–206

34. Oliver C, Holland AJ (1986) Down's syndrome and Alzheimer's disease: a review. Psychol Med 16: 307–322

35. Olson L, Backlund E-O, Ebendal T, Freedman R, Hamberger B, Hansson P, Hoffer B, Lindblom U, Meyerson B, Strömberg I,

Sydow O, Seiger Å (1991) Intraputaminal infusion of nerve growth factor to support adrenal medullary autografts in Parkinson's disease. Arch Neurol 48: 373–381

36. Pearson RCA, Powell TPS (1989) The neuroanatomy of Alzheimer's disease. Rev Neurosci 2: 101–122

37. Perry EK (1986) The cholinergic hypothesis – ten years on. Br Med Bull 42: 63–69

38. Perry EK, Tomlinson BE, Blessed G, Bergmann K, Gibson PH, Perry RH (1978) Correlation of cholinergic abnormalities with senile plaques and mental test scores in senile dementia. Br Med J ii: 1457–1459

39. Quon D, Wang Y, Catalano R, Marian Scardina J, Murakami K, Cordell B (1991) Formation of β-amyloid protein deposits in brains of transgenic mice. Nature 352: 239–241

40. Richards S-J (1991) The neuropathology of Alzheimer's disease investigated by transplantation of mouse trisomy 16 hippocampal tissues. Trends Neurosci 14: 334–338

41. Richards S-J, Waters JJ, Abraham CJ, Sparkman DR, White CL, Beyreuther K, Masters CL, Dunnett SB (1991) Transplants of mouse trisomy 16 hippocampus provide an in vivo model of the neuropathology of Alzheimer's disease. EMBO J 10: 297–303

42. Richter-Levin G, Segal M (1989) Raphe cells grafted into the hippocampus can ameliorate spatial memory deficits in rats with combined serotonergic/cholinergic deficiencies. Brain Res 478: 184–186

43. Ridley RM, Baker HF (1991) Can fetal neural transplants restore function in monkeys with lesion-induced behavioural deficits? Trends Neurosci 14: 366–370

44. Rosenberg MB, Friedmann T, Robertson RC, Tuszynski M, Wolff JA, Breakefield XO, Gage FH (1988) Grafting of genetically modified cells to the damaged brain: restorative effects of NGF expression. Science 242: 1575–1578

45. Sofroniew MV, Pearson RCA (1985) Degeneration of cholinergic neurons in the basal nucleus following kainic acid or N-methyl-D-aspartic acid application to the cerebral cortex in the rat. Brain Res 339: 186–190

46. Sofroniew MV, Isacson O, Björklund A (1986) Cortical grafts prevent atrophy of cholinergic basal nucleus neurons induced by excitotoxic cortical damage. Brain Res 378: 409–415

47. Sofroniew MV, Dunnett SB, Isacson O (1990) Remodelling of intrinsic and afferent systems during loss and replacement of cortical neurons. Prog Brain Res 82: 313–320

48. Springer JE, Collier TJ, Sladek JR, Loy R (1988) Transplantation of male mouse submaxillary gland increases survival of axotomised basal forebrain neurons. J Neurosci Res 19: 291–296

49. Stoll J, Ault B, Rapoport SI, Fine A (1991) Examination of Alzheimer-type pathology in mouse trisomy 16 neurons maintained by transplantation. Soc Neurosci Abstr 17: 1064

50. Tomlinson BE, Corsellis JAN (1984) Aging and the dementias. In: Hume Adams J, Corsellis JAN, Duchen IW (eds) Greenfield's neuropathology. Wiley, New York, pp 951–1025

51. Tomlinson BE, Blessed G, Roth M (1970) Observations on the brains of demented old people. J Neurol Sci 11: 205–242

52. Vanderwolf CH (1987) Near-total loss of "learning" and "memory" as a result of combined cholinergic and serotonergic blockade in the rat. Behav Brain Res 23: 43–57

53. Wischik CM, Novak M, Thorensen HC, Edwards PC, Runswick MJ, Jakes R, Walker JE, Milstein C, Roth M, Klug A (1988) Isolation of a fragment of tau derived from the core of the paired helical filament of Alzheimer's disease. Proc Natl Acad Sci USA 85: 4506–4510

54. Yamaguchi F, Richards SJ, Beyreuther K, Dunnett SB (1991) Transgenic mice for the amyloid precursor protein 695 isoform show spatial memory impairment. NeuroReport 2: 781–784

Transplantation in Experimental Epilepsy

J. Bengzon and O. Lindvall

Restorative Neurology Unit, Department of Neurology, University Hospital, Lund, Sweden

Introduction

Epileptic seizures are characterized by hyperexcitability and synchrony among populations of central neurons, but the mechanisms underlying the abnormal patterns of electric activity are only partly known. There is evidence from human autopsy material that the increased excitability results from a loss of inhibitory, presumably GABA-ergic, neurons (GABA, γ-aminobutyric acid). Possibly the hyperexcitability also depends on an abnormal increase of excitatory synaptic mechanisms. Finally, at least in experimental animals, some long-loop neuronal circuitries might be able to influence the development and generalization of epileptiform activity; for example, the noradrenergic locus ceruleus system, which originates in the pons and has widespread projections to almost the entire CNS, dampens seizures in the brain.

Compared with studies on models of neurodegenerative diseases, considerably less work has been done with neural grafts in experimental epilepsy. One major explanation is that, unlike the situation for instance in Parkinson's disease, the deficit in epilepsy that should be corrected by grafts has not been identified. Furthermore, several models of epilepsy are unsuitable for intracerebral grafting (ICG) experiments: some give rise to epileptic syndromes that are either too variable or transient and resolve before the graft-derived innervation is complete, and others require the use of a seizure-inducing agent that is toxic to the transplanted fetal neurons.

Most ICG studies in experimental epilepsy have used fetal tissue from the locus ceruleus region rich in norepinephrine (NE), for a number of reasons. First, considerable evidence indicated that intrinsic locus ceruleus neurons dampen epileptic activity in the CNS (see, for instance, [12]); second, the anatomy of this system is well known, and the locus ceruleus neurons can easily be demonstrated microscopically or destroyed with relative specificity by the neurotoxin 6-hydroxydopamine (6-OHDA; see, for instance, [7]); third, there is an extensive knowledge of the biochemical, pharmacologic, and physiologic characteristics of pre- and postsynaptic noradrenergic mechanisms (see, for instance, [18]); and fourth, grafted locus ceruleus neurons have been shown to grow into the host brain and to modify the function and behavior of the host (see, for instance, [31]).

The present chapter will show how neuronal grafting has been used as a tool to reduce neuronal excitability and has provided interesting data on the pathophysiologic mechanisms involved in experimental seizures. The main emphasis will be on the ICG of noradrenergic locus ceruleus neurons, but also studies using other types of donor tissue will be summarized. Finally, some current research strategies and possible future clinical developments will be discussed.

Noradrenergic Grafts in Experimental Epilepsy

Hippocampal Kindling in NE-Depleted Forebrain

Kindling is one of the most extensively studied animal models of epilepsy (see, for instance, [41]): repeated administration of an initially subconvulsive electric stimulus results in progressive intensification of stimulus-induced seizure activity, culminating in a generalized seizure. The initial stimulus evokes focal seizure activity (so-called afterdischarge) in the EEG without there being clinical signs of convulsions. Subsequent stimulations lead to the development of kindled behavioral seizures, which generally proceed through five grades [40] (Fig. 1). An animal that has exhibited grade 5 seizures is said to be kindled. This effect is permanent: even if the animal is left unstimulated for as long as 12 months, it will respond to one of the first electric stimuli with a grade 5 seizure [48]. Kindling triggered by stimulation in the limbic system has been proposed to be analogous to partial epilepsy with complex symptomatology, also called temporal lobe epilepsy [33], which is the most frequent type of epilepsy in adult humans [20].

Rats with extensive lesions of the NE neurons in the forebrain induced by the intraventricular injection of 6-OHDA exhibit a marked acceleration of the rate of kindling evoked by electric stimulation in the amygdala or hippocampus. This is due to the removal of the powerful inhibitory influence on the development of kindled seizures normally exerted by the locus ceruleus system [31].

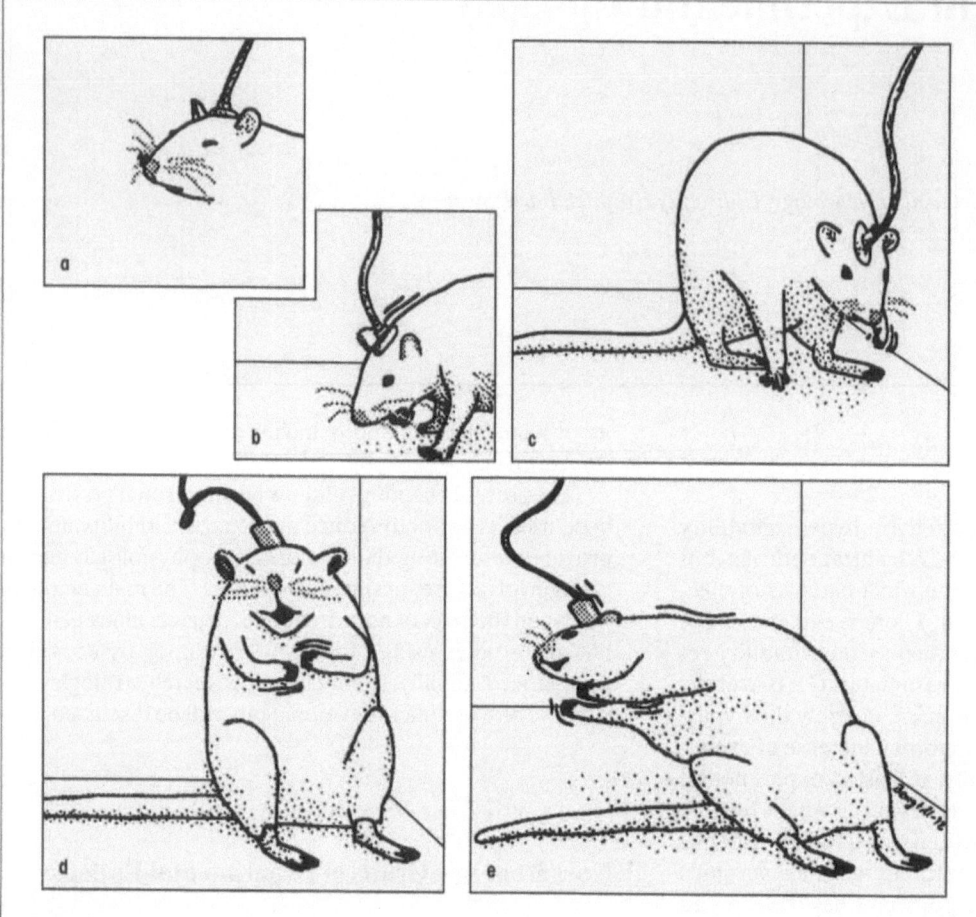

Fig. 1. *Seizure development in the kindling model of epilepsy. Intensification and lengthening of electroencephalographic seizure activity is accompanied by behavioral seizures that can be divided into five grades of increasing severity:* **a**, *facial twitches;* **b**, *head nodding;* **c**, *forelimb clonus;* **d**, *rearing;* **e**, *rearing and falling*

Intracerebral transplantation experiments have been carried out in such animals with the main objectives, first, of finding out whether locus ceruleus grafts can reverse the functional deficit induced by 6-OHDA and retard the kindling rate in NE-depleted, hyperexcitable rats; second, of finding out the functional mode of action of these grafts; and, third, of obtaining more information on the role and mode of action of the intrinsic locus ceruleus system in kindled animals. Locus ceruleus grafts implanted bilaterally into the hippocampus retarded the development of hippocampal kindling in NE-depleted rats (Fig. 2a and b) [1]. The NE neurons in the grafts had reinnervated the dorsal two-thirds of the hippocampal formation, whereas only few graft-derived NE axons were observed outside the hippocampus (Fig. 2c and d). This indicates that the reinstatement of NE transmission at the kindling site (corresponding to the epileptic focus) is sufficient to suppress seizure development even in these extensively denervated animals. The retardation of kindling was significantly correlated with the degree of noradrenergic axonal ingrowth from the graft into the host hippocampus, a fact supporting the view that the seizure-suppressant action of the grafts was mediated by NE mechanisms. Furthermore, the dampening action of intrahippocampal locus ceruleus grafts could be blocked by the systemic administration of the α_2-adrenergic receptor

antagonist idazoxan (Fig. 3) [5]. This may suggest [21] that NE released from the grafts influences the kindling rate through activation of postsynaptic α_2-adrenergic receptors.

The functional capacity of locus ceruleus grafts has also been tested after implantation in a region distant from the stimulating electrode [2]. The amygdala-piriform cortex was chosen as the implantation site since this region has been proposed to be of central importance for the development and expression of kindled seizures [32, 41]. Locus ceruleus grafts, which probably reinstated NE transmission bilaterally in the amygdala-piriform cortex, retarded the rate of kindling evoked by hippocampal stimulation to the same degree as if they had been implanted in the hippocampus (Fig. 2b). Thus, implants in a restricted region of critical importance for the spread and generalization of seizures could influence the susceptibility to seizures in widespread areas of the CNS including the epileptic focus.

Much information on how locus ceruleus grafts exert their seizure-suppressant effects has been obtained by means of intracerebral microdialysis to monitor the release of NE during and between seizures (Fig. 4a, b). There is good evidence that the extracellular NE levels in the dialysis perfusate are derived from neurons and can be used as indices of noradrenergic synaptic activity. The steady-state NE output in the hippocampus of animal graft recipients

Fig. 2. *a* Dorsal view of the CNS of a rat on embryonic day 13 (crown-rump length, 12 mm). The tectum has been cut midsagittally and folded back to expose the floor of the fourth ventricle. The **shaded area** indicates the dissected pontine tissue containing the locus ceruleus neuroblast. **CB**, cerebellar bud; **LC**, locus ceruleus; **PF**, pontine flexure; **T**, tectum; **TV**, telencephalic vesicle. (Modified from [9]).

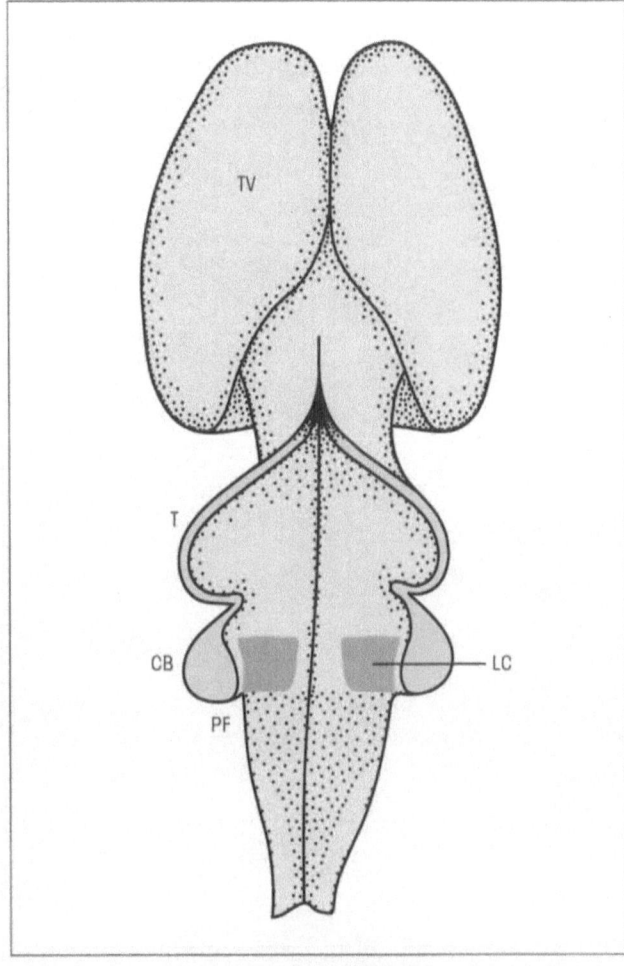

Fig. 2. *b* Number of hippocampal kindling stimulations required to reach grade 1 and grade 5 seizures in 6-OHDA-treated, NE-depleted rats (lesioned rats), in 6-OHDA-treated animals with bilateral grafts of fetal locus ceruleus in either the amygdala-piriform cortex (grafted rats, **left part** of diagram) or the hippocampus (grafted rats, **right part** of diagram), and in animals with an intact noradrenergic innervation (controls). Seizures developed more slowly in graft recipients than in other lesioned rats, but the kindling rate in the group with intrahippocampal grafts was still facilitated in comparison with controls. Graft recipients are significantly different from lesioned animals without grafts (*) and from intact controls (+) (Modified from [2]).

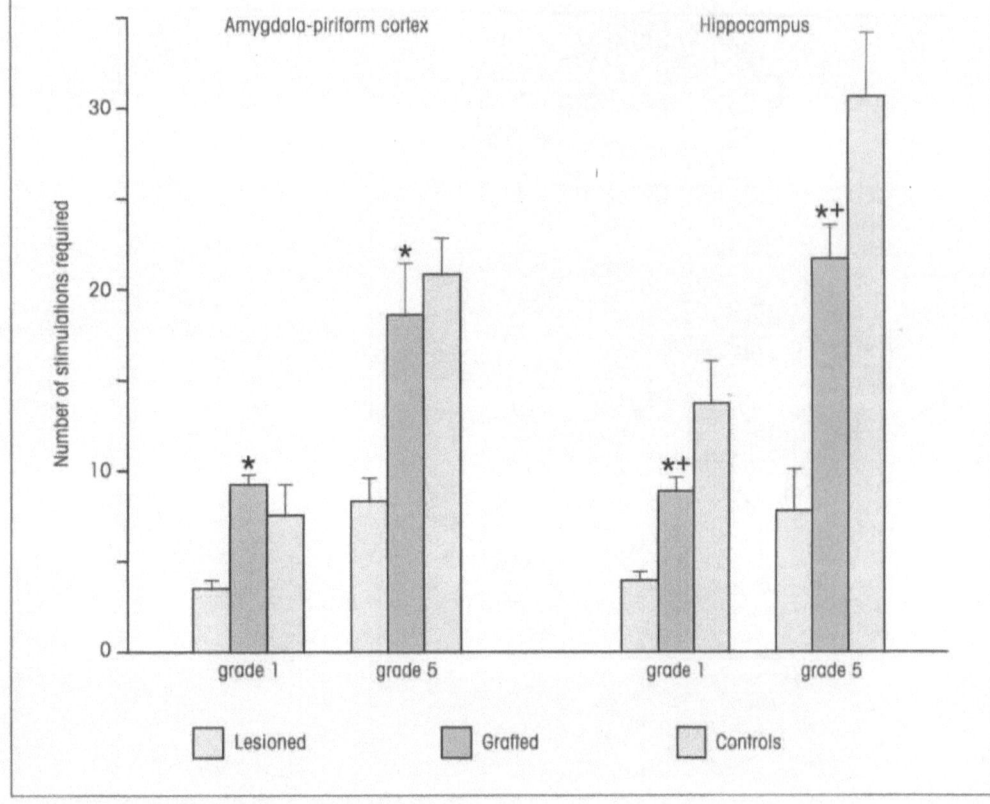

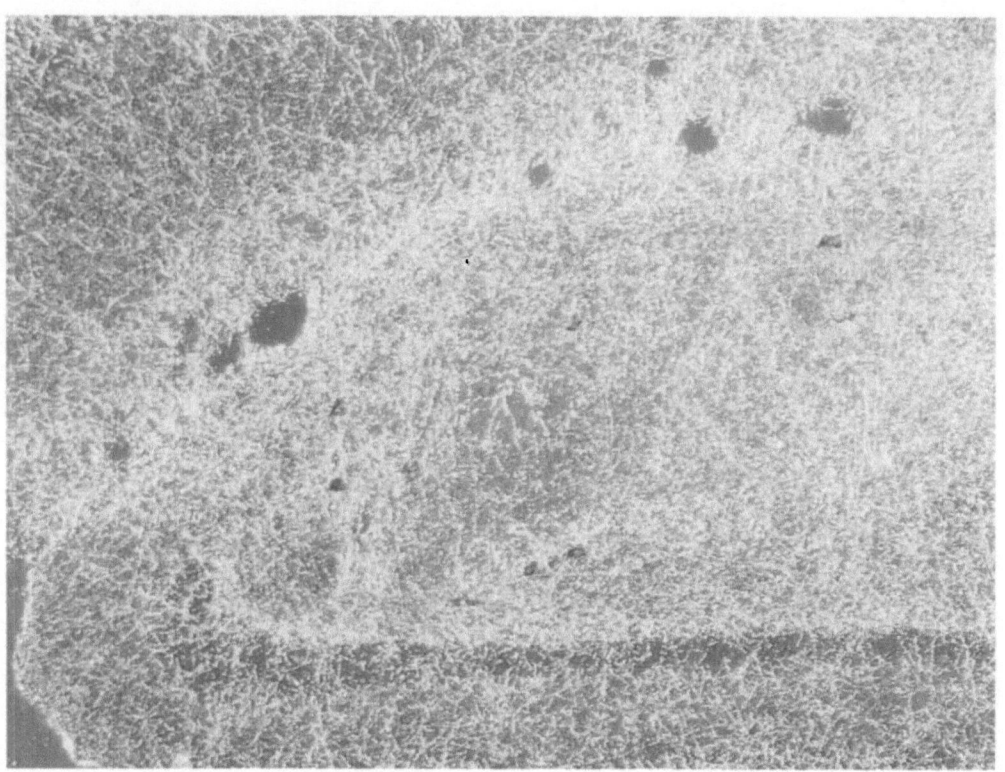

Fig. 2. c Dark-field photomicrograph of grafted neurons and fibers in the dentate gyrus of a previously 6-OHDA-treated, NE-depleted rat; immunostaining for dopamine β-hydroxylase.

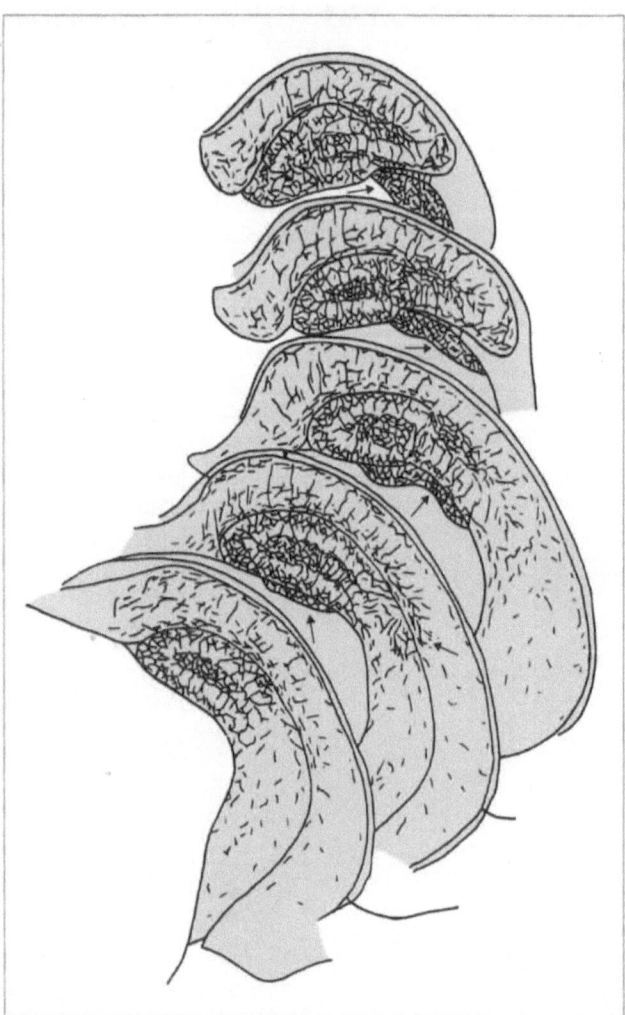

Fig. 2. d Schematic illustration of selected serial sections at different rostrocaudal levels within the same animal, showing the noradrenergic innervation produced by a seizure-suppressant graft of fetal locus ceruleus tissue in the hippocampus rendered hyperexcitable by denervation. The arrows indicate the location of the graft. (Modified from [1])

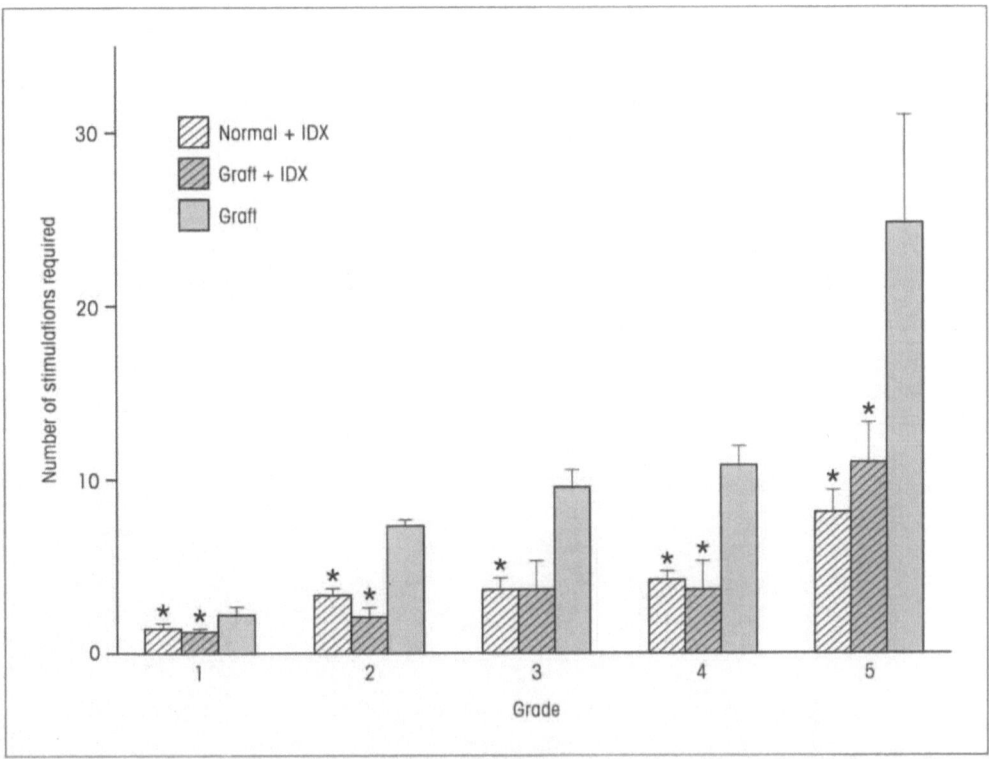

Fig. 3. Progression of hippocampal kindling in normal rats or NE-depleted rats with bilateral grafts of locus ceruleus tissue to the hippocampus. The α-adrenoceptor blocker idazoxan (**IDX**) was administered before every stimulation in the normal group and in one of the two groups of animals with grafts. * Significantly different from rats not treated with IDX. (Modified from [5])

previously denervated with 6-OHDA was similar to the baseline output in normal rats [3]. A generalized seizure of about 2 min duration gave rise to a severalfold increase of hippocampal NE levels in both normal animals and graft recipients (Fig. 4b). The maximal increase of NE output occurred within 2–4 min after the onset of seizure activity, and the extracellular levels then tapered off, reaching baseline values after another 6–8 min. Microdialysis experiments performed during seizures before and after acute transection of the ascending axons from the locus ceruleus indicated [3, 4] that the increased NE output evoked by epileptic activity is dependent on impulse flow in locus ceruleus neurons and probably also on local regulatory mechanisms acting at the noradrenergic terminal level. These findings are in agreement with the increased firing rate found in intrinsic locus ceruleus neurons during kindled seizures [24].

From the microdialysis experiments it can be concluded that epileptic seizures are associated with a temporally defined, well-regulated increase in NE output from both intrinsic and grafted locus ceruleus neurons occurring concurrently with their seizure-suppressant action. Despite their ectopic location in the hippocampus, the grafted locus ceruleus neurons seem to be functionally integrated with the host brain, at least during generalized kindled seizures. In the denervated hippocampus, locus ceruleus grafts form a noradrenergic terminal plexus that is very similar to the one seen in the intact brain. They establish synaptic contacts with host hippocampal neurons and also seem to be innervated by the host [35]. This afferent input, the origin of

which is not known, may mediate the regulatory influence of the recipient's brain on NE release from the graft in response to seizures.

Spontaneous and Picrotoxin-Induced Seizures in Animals with Subcortical Hippocampus Denervation

Another epilepsy model suitable for ICG experiments is created by removing major parts of the subcortical inhibitory input to the hippocampus [10]. The lesion involves aspiration of the medial portion of the parietal cortex and cingulate cortex and transects the cingulate bundle, the supracallosal stria, the corpus callosum, the dorsal fornix, the fimbria, and the ventral hippocampal commissure (Fig. 5a). According to Buszáki et al. [10], this leads to the removal of cholinergic and GABA-ergic afferents from the septal area, noradrenergic afferents from the locus ceruleus, serotoninergic efferents from the mesencephalic raphe, several other minor pathways from other subcortical nuclei, the commissural pathways, and the subcortical efferent projection of the hippocampal formation.

Animals with this lesion show increased susceptibility to behavioral seizures induced by picrotoxin (a GABA-receptor antagonist) and a higher frequency of interictal spikes in the hippocampus both before and after repeated hippocampal seizures evoked by electric stimulation of the perforant path (Fig. 5b) [10]. Grafts of fetal locus ceruleus tissue implanted bilaterally into the hippocampus of lesioned ani-

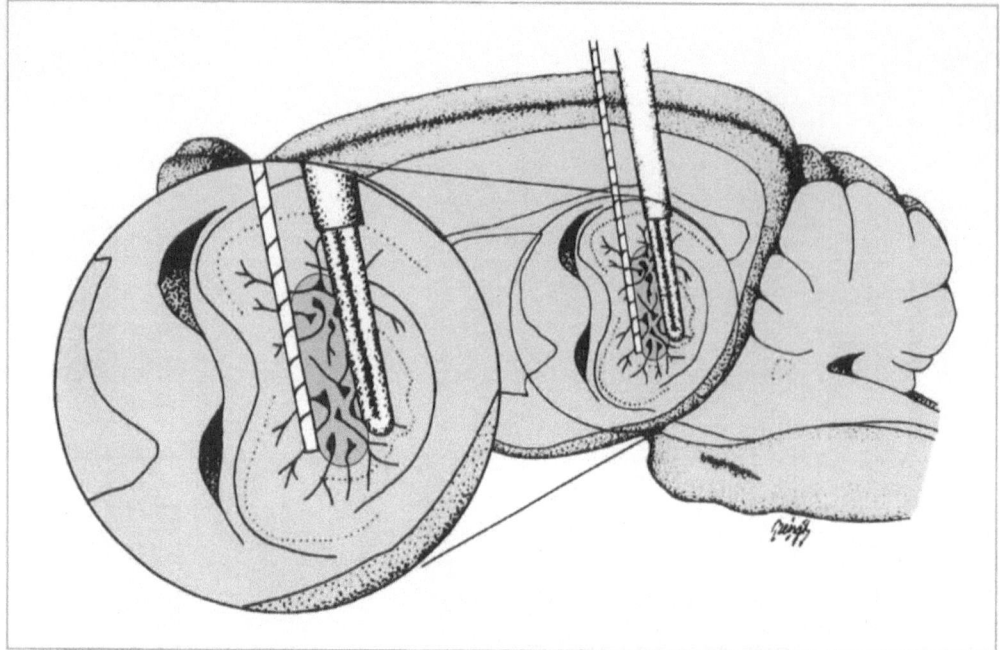

Fig. 4. a *Location of the stimulating/recording electrode and microdialysis probe next to the locus ceruleus graft in the hippocampal formation.*

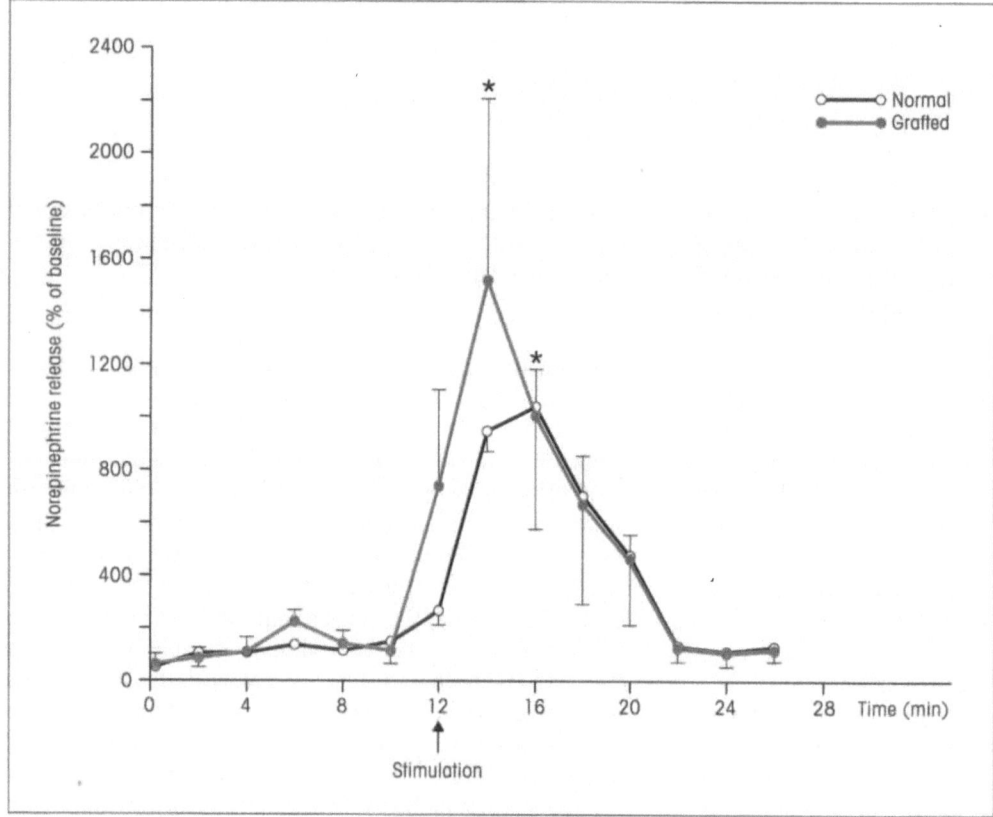

Fig. 4. b *NE release in the hippocampus in response to a generalized kindled seizure lasting about 2 min in normal rats and 6-OHDA-treated, NE-depleted rats with locus ceruleus grafts in the hippocampus. The NE uptake blocker desipramine was continuously present in the perfusion fluid.*
* Significantly different from the preceding baseline level. (Modified from [3])

mals reduced the incidence of interictal spikes in the host hippocampus and protected against picrotoxin-induced behavioral seizures (Fig. 5b). Control grafts consisting of fetal hippocampal tissue had the opposite effect. The locus ceruleus grafts contained noradrenergic neurons from which axonal processes extended into the host hippocampus. Buszáki et al. [10] proposed that the grafted locus ceruleus neurons may have influenced seizure susceptibility in this model either through a direct action of NE on hippocampal pyramidal cells or by competing with sprouting axons of host neurons for postsynaptic sites that had become vacant after the lesion, thereby limiting excessive collateral excitation.

Fig. 5. a Schematic view of the
aspiration lesion used to create a
hyperexcitable hippocampus
through subcortical denervation.
The lesion involves, for instance,
the medial parietal and cingulate
cortices, the corpus callosum,
and dorsal fornix and fimbria.
The septal cholinergic neurons,
indicated in the drawing,
represent one of the many
subcortical afferent projections
to the hippocampus that are
transected by the lesion. Also
shown is a locus ceruleus
transplant to the hippocampus.

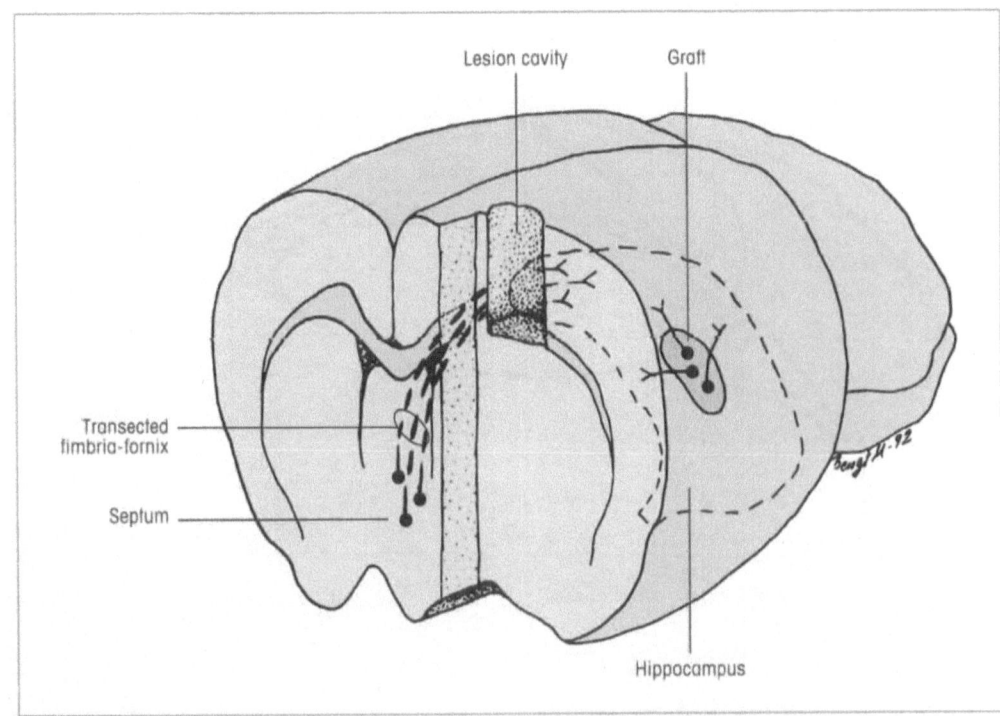

Fig. 5. b Interictal spike
frequency in the hippocampus
1 day before (*yellow columns*)
and 1 day after (*blue columns*)
six seizures induced by perforant
path stimulation in rats with
lesions of the fimbria-fornix
(*FF*) as illustrated in Fig. 5 a and
in animals with fimbria-fornix
lesions and intrahippocampal
grafts of fetal hippocampus
(*HPC*) or locus ceruleus (*LC*).
*Significantly different from
intact and LC groups. (Modified
from [10])*

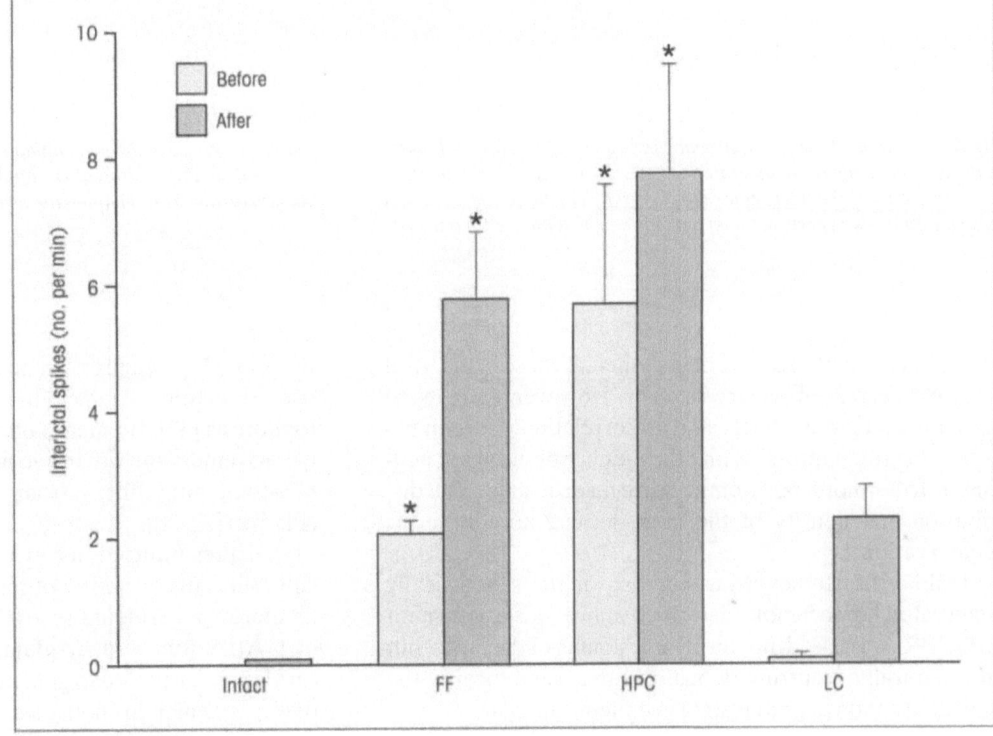

Audiogenic Seizures in Genetically Epilepsy-Prone Rats

Genetically epilepsy-prone rats (GEPRs) exhibit a lack of
seizure-suppressing mechanisms, including a deficit in noradrenergic transmission. GEPRs have lower levels and
turnover rates of NE, reduced high-affinity NE uptake and
dopamine-β-hydroxylase activity, and fewer nerve terminals in the forebrain and several other CNS regions than
controls [8, 25, 28, 29]. Fetal NE-rich locus ceruleus tissue
has, in a preliminary study [13], been implanted into
GEPRs to elucidate whether restoration of noradrenergic
transmission by the grafts may reduce the severity of audio-
genic seizures evoked by a bell tone. The implantation site
was either the hippocampus or the third ventricle. Hip-

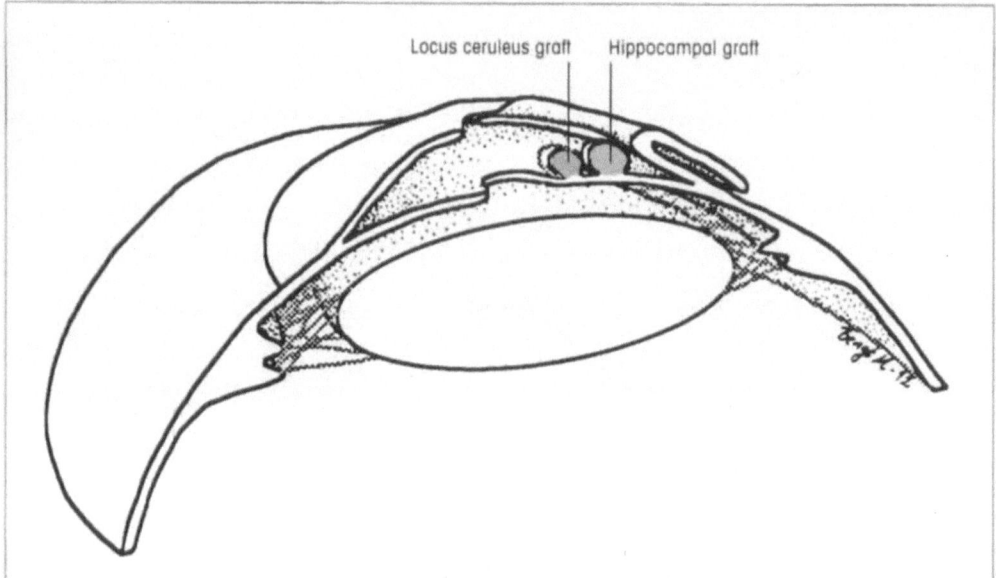

Fig. 6. a *Schematic representation of double grafts of fetal hippocampus and locus ceruleus tissue to the anterior chamber of the eye.*

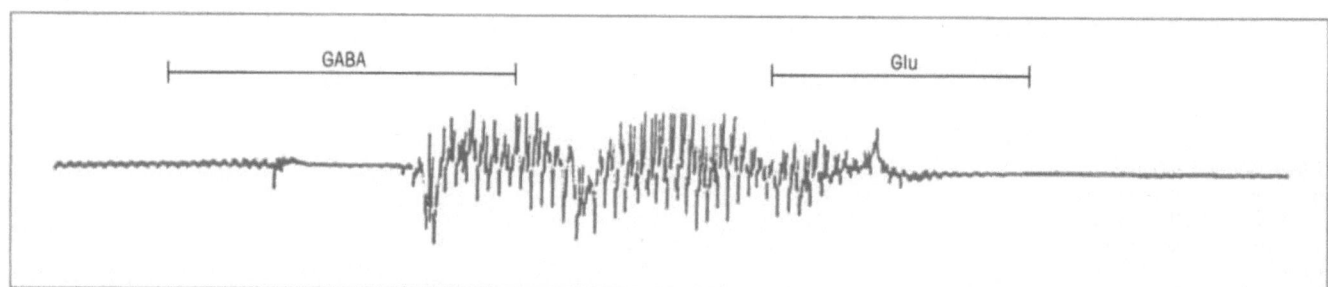

Fig. 6. b *Effects of the iontophoretic application of GABA and gluta-mate into the locus ceruleus graft on the EEG recorded from the hip-pocampal part of the intraocular double graft. The hippocampus graft was continuously superfused with penicillin, which induced seizure ac-tivity in response to the concomitant iontophoresis of GABA into the lo-cus ceruleus graft. Subsequent application of glutamate into the locus ceruleus graft terminated seizure activity. (Modified from [47])*

pocampal implants had no effects, whereas those in the third ventricle decreased seizure severity. However, there were no significant group effects, and no correlation was seen be-tween seizure suppression and the number of surviving neu-rons. Furthermore, no attempts were made to assess the dis-tribution and density of the graft-derived noradrenergic reinnervation.

Unlike the studies using kindling or the subcortically denervated hippocampus described above, this experiment on GEPRs was based, not on prior lesioning of the brain, but on a naturally occurring deficit and thus came nearer the clinical situation of graft testing in epileptic humans.

Penicillin-Induced Seizures in Fetal Hippocampus Tissue Implanted in the Eye

Pieces of fetal hippocampus placed on the iris in the anterior chamber of the eye in adult rats grow and develop a laminar neuronal organization. Also intrinsic excitatory and in-hibitory circuitries typical of the hippocampus in situ form in the graft [36]. Seizures can be induced in such grafts by elec-tric stimulation, penicillin superfusion, and cobalt ion-tophoresis [22]. By means of sequential grafting, it is possi-ble to innervate an intraocular hippocampal graft with NE-containing fibers from a locus ceruleus transplant (Fig. 6a) [37, 38].

Seizures induced in single hippocampal grafts by peni-cillin superfusion were not seen in the presence of cografts of fetal locus ceruleus tissue (Fig. 6b) [47]. Local application of GABA followed by glutamate onto the grafted locus ceruleus neurons led to generation and suppression, respec-tively, of penicillin-induced epileptiform activity in the hip-pocampus graft (Fig. 6b). This suggested that a functional inhibitory innervation had developed between the locus ceruleus graft and neurons in the hippocampus graft. The in-hibitory influence was blocked by reserpine, a fact support-ing the involvement of noradrenergic mechanisms.

Further support for the seizure-suppressant action of NE in this model was obtained in experiments in which sym-pathetic adrenergic fibers from the host iris reinnervated single hippocampal grafts [19]. Electric stimulation of the cervical sympathetic trunk activating these noradrenergic afferents reduced both the amplitude and the frequency of penicillin-induced epileptiform activity. This effect could be blocked by a β-adrenergic receptor antagonist.

Other Grafts in Experimental Epilepsy

Serotoninergic Neurons

Kindling epilepsy can be induced also by electric stimulation of the olfactory bulb. Although the role of the serotoninergic system in kindling evoked from other structures, e.g., the amygdala and the hippocampus, is unclear, serotoninergic afferents seem to inhibit kindling in the olfactory bulb [30]. Specific neurotoxin-induced lesions of the olfactory bulb's serotoninergic innervation lead to facilitation of seizure development in kindling. By analogy with the experiments described above in which NE-rich tissue from the locus ceruleus region was implanted in the NE-depleted hippocampus, 5-hydroxytryptamine-(5-HT-)rich fetal tissue from the raphe region has been grafted into the olfactory bulbs of adult rats previously depleted of 5-HT by means of 5,7-dihydroxytryptamine injections. In other studies, intrahippocampal raphe grafts have reinnervated the denervated hippocampus and restored the levels and release of 5-HT [14, 15]. Also in the olfactory bulb the grafted serotoninergic neurons exhibited extensive axonal outgrowth. The raphe grafts reversed the facilitatory effect on the development of olfactory bulb kindling caused by the neurotoxin lesion [11].

GABA-ergic Neurons

So far, there has been no conclusive experimental evidence that the ICG of GABA-rich tissue can influence epileptic activity. Stevens et al. [46] reported that grafts of fetal cerebellar or cortical tissue placed in the deep prepiriform area of amygdala-kindled rats, i. e., grafts intended to provide the host brain with additional GABA neurons at a site important for seizure generalization, transiently raised the seizure thresholds in only a minority of animals. Furthermore, no presumably GABA-ergic neurons immunopositive for glutamic acid decarboxylase (GAD) could be demonstrated in the graft.

Another model used for the ICG of GABA-rich tissue is created by systemic administration of the muscarinic cholinergic agonist pilocarpine to rats (references in [17]). The resulting seizures are considered to resemble complex partial epilepsy in humans. Susceptibility to such pilocarpine-induced seizures is increased by lesions of the strionigral GABA-ergic projection caused by neurotoxin injections in the caudate-putamen. Transplantation of GABA-rich tissue from the fetal striatum into the substantia nigra attenuated the lesion-induced increase in seizure susceptibility

[17]. However, in this study no attempt was made to assess the degree of survival of GABA-ergic neurons in the graft. Furthermore, the control grafts consisting of sciatic nerve had the same effects on seizure susceptibility as the implants of striatal tissue. Thus, the functional effects observed after ICG could not be attributed to an increased GABA-ergic inhibition provided by the grafts.

Present Lines of Research and Clinical Perspectives

From the clinical point of view, it seems highly warranted to explore further to what extent grafts can suppress the generation, spread, severity, and duration of convulsive activity in the epileptic brain. The principal strategy underlying the ICG approach seems very simple, i. e., to reduce neuronal hyperexcitability in an epileptic brain region by implanting cells that have an inhibitory effect. The further progress of this research is, however, complicated by two major problems. First, no deficit in a particular transmitter system has been shown to underlie most forms of experimental or clinical epilepsy; this is in contrast to the situation in Parkinson's disease, where the ICG of neural tissue aims at restoring dopamine synthesis, storage, and release at synaptic sites through a reinnervation of the striatum by grafted mesencephalic dopaminergic neurons. Second, it is largely unknown whether the addition of "inhibitory" neurons to an epileptic brain region without a deficit in that particular neuron system leads to increased inhibition. For example, to what extent are implanted GABA-producing cells anatomically and functionally integrated with the host brain? These cells, rather than suppress seizures, might cause increased excitation as their resultant functional action, particularly when placed at an ectopic site.

At present it seems most appropriate to focus on the ICG of tissue rich in either NE- or GABA-producing cells, which appear to be the ones most suitable for reducing neuronal hyperexcitability. In the following paragraphs, some important issues related to the use of NE- or GABA-producing cells will be discussed.

Norepinephrine-Producing Grafts

Three main problems should be addressed:
1. Can NE-producing cells suppress convulsions, i. e., inhibit epileptic activity, when implanted in animals with a fully developed epileptic syndrome? In previous kindling experiments [1, 2], the neurons were grafted before the start of stimulations, and in the subcortically denervated animals [10] cell implantation took place about 1 week after the fornix-fimbria lesion. In both models, the influence of locus ceruleus grafts might be regarded as primarily antiepileptogenic rather than anticonvulsant, i. e., they counteracted the development of hyperexcitability while

having no effect on established seizures. If locus ceruleus neurons are implanted bilaterally into the hippocampus in 6-OHDA-denervated animals after kindling is established, no effects on the duration and severity of seizures are observed [6]. These findings argue against an anticonvulsant action of grafted locus ceruleus neurons in kindling epilepsy. However, an anticonvulsant effect cannot yet be totally excluded, since it may require graft-derived innervations in widespread areas outside the hippocampus and/or in regions critical for seizure generalization.

2. Can NE-rich grafts reduce neuronal excitability after implantation into a region without prior lesion-induced denervation of the intrinsic noradrenergic input? Implantation of locus ceruleus neurons into the nondenervated hippocampus leads to a noradrenergic hyperinnervation, and the grafted noradrenergic cells seem to form synaptic contacts with host hippocampal neurons [35]. This extra NE input, however, does not influence the seizure development in kindling, i.e., it has no antiepileptogenic effect [6]. When implanted into intact, kindled animals, the grafts increase both the basal and the seizure-evoked NE release in the stimulated hippocampus [6], but it is unknown whether this increase leads to any change in neuronal excitability within the area of the hippocampus innervated by the graft. The experimental situation is comparable in some respects to that when locus ceruleus neurons are grafted to genetically epilepsy-prone animals: the intrinsic NE system is present even though there are functional impairments [8, 25, 28, 29].

3. Is the seizure-depressant effect of grafted NE-producing cells dependent on NE release at synaptic sites and functional integration with the host brain? If so, genetically engineered nonneuronal cells, cell lines enclosed in polymer capsules, or adrenal medulla cells, even though able to provide NE and other catecholamines, would probably not be capable of dampening epileptic activity. On the other hand, if a more diffuse, hormonal, and less finely regulated release of NE is sufficient, these various cell types might constitute useful alternatives to fetal neurons.

GABA-Producing Grafts

A major problem with increasing GABA-ergic transmission within a brain region by means of neural grafts has consisted in finding a suitable source of GABA-rich tissue. Although GABA neurons from the striatum can survive both in the normal and the kainic-acid-treated epileptic hippocampus, the grafts are often small and poorly integrated with the host brain ([43] and unpublished observations). This contrasts with grafts placed in the striatum, where they form extensive afferent and efferent connections with the host brain [49–51] and release GABA [44]. Other possible sources of GABA neurons such as the fetal substantia nigra or cerebellum should be tested, but grafts from these regions will probably yield inadequate results too when implanted at ectopic sites. Enriched GABA-ergic neurons, prepared by cell sorting, could represent one future alternative. Another attrac-

tive possibility may be the ICG of genetically engineered GABA-producing cells; in the case of nonneuronal cells, it remains to be established – as for the NE cells discussed above – whether nonsynaptic GABA release is sufficient for a seizure-supressant action to be exerted and whether some degree of regulation of the graft by the host brain is required.

Available experimental evidence suggests that GABA-producing cells might influence epileptic phenomena after implantation in at least two entirely different sites. First, they may be effective when implanted in the epileptic focus, where according to some reports there is a deficit of GABA-ergic transmission, e.g., after hippocampal kindling [26, 27] or the application of cobalt [16] or alumina cream [42]. However, the grafting of GABA cells to the epileptic focus might, even if there is no deficit in intrinsic GABA-ergic transmission, counteract hyperexcitability due to perturbations in other neuronal systems. Second, grafts might prove effective when implanted in regions of importance for the generalization of epileptic seizures. One such site is the pars reticularis of the substantia nigra; bilateral microinjections of GABA agonists into this region suppress electroconvulsive shock seizures [23] and chemically induced seizures [23] as well as kindled seizures [34]. A similar functional effect could possibly be exerted also by GABA-producing cells implanted into the substantia nigra. Another critical region that might be suitable for the transplantation of GABA neurons is the area tempesta in the deep prepiriform area [39]. Infusion of a GABA agonist or a transaminase inhibitor into this region has been shown to suppress both chemically induced and kindled seizures [39, 45]. As described above, there have been a few, largely negative, attempts at implanting GABA-rich tissue in the substantia nigra and the deep prepiriform region [17, 46].

Concluding Remarks

The use of ICG as an investigative tool in epilepsy research is still in its infancy. The potential value of this approach, however, is already shown by evidence that neural grafts can suppress epileptic phenomena in the CNS. Further studies should elucidate to what extent different components of the epileptic syndrome can be influenced by cell implants. For example, can grafts have both antiepileptogenic and anticonvulsant effects? Where should grafts be placed – in the epileptic focus, in regions of critical importance for seizure generalization, or at multiple sites in order to innervate large volumes of the epileptic brain? The mechanism of action of grafts in epilepsy should also be further explored. Do the grafts have to act via a controlled synaptic release of transmitter, or is a biologic minipump delivering the compound in a more diffuse, hormonal manner sufficient? What level of anatomic and functional integration into the host neuronal circuitry is necessary for grafts to modulate neuronal excitability and convulsive phenomena? Obviously, general advances in the field of ICG will have a direct impact on its use in epilepsy research, e. g., the production of genetically engineered cells making possible the implantation of a pure population producing a single transmitter such as GABA. This research will conceivably provide new insights into the pathophysiology of seizures and, it is to be hoped, the necessary basis for attempting to reduce neuronal hyperexcitability in human epilepsy by means of the ICG of cells.

Acknowledgements. Our own research reviewed here was supported by grants from the Swedish Medical Research Council (14X–8666), the Thorsten and Elsa Segerfalk Foundation, and the Bank of Sweden Tricentenary Fund. We are grateful to Gerd Andersson for valuable secretarial help.

References

1. Barry DI, Kikvadze I, Brundin P, Bolwig TG, Björklund A, Lindvall O (1987) Grafted noradrenergic neurons suppress seizure development in kindling-induced epilepsy. Proc Natl Acad Sci USA 84: 8712–8715

2. Barry DI, Wanscher B, Kragh J, Bolwig TG, Kokaia M, Brundin P, Björklund A, Lindvall O (1989) Grafts of fetal locus coeruleus neurons in rat amygdala-piriform cortex suppress seizure development in hippocampal kindling. Exp Neurol 106: 125–132

3. Bengzon J, Brundin P, Kalen P, Kokaia M, Lindvall O (1991) Host regulation of noradrenaline release from grafts of seizure-suppressant locus coeruleus neurons. Exp Neurol 111: 49–54

4. Bengzon J, Kikvadze I, Kokaia M, Lindvall O (1992) Regional forebrain noradrenaline release in response to focal and generalized seizures induced by hippocampal kindling stimulation. Eur J Neurosci 4: 278–288

5. Bengzon J, Kokaia M, Brundin P, Lindvall O (1990) Seizure suppression in kindling epilepsy by intrahippocampal locus coeruleus grafts: evidence for an alpha₂-adrenoreceptor mediated mechanism. Exp Brain Res 81: 433–437

6. Bengzon J, Kokaia Z, Lindvall O'(1993) Specific functions of grafted locus coeruleus neurons in the kindling model of epilepsy. Exp Neurol (in press)

7. Björklund A, Lindvall O (1986) Catecholaminergic brain stem regulatory systems. In: Bloom FE (ed) Handbook of physiology – the nervous system: IV. Intrinsic regulatory system in the brain. American Physiological Society, Bethesda; pp 155–235

8. Browning RA, Wade DR, Marcinczyk M, Long GL, Jobe PC (1989) Regional brain abnormalities in norepinephrine uptake and dopamine beta-hydroxylase activity in the genetically epilepsy-prone rat. J Pharmacol Exp Ther 249: 229–235

9. Brundin P, Strecker A (1991) Preparation and intracerebral grafting of dissociated fetal brain tissue in rats. In: Conn PM (ed) Lesions and transplantation. Academic, San Diego, pp 305–326 (Methods in neurosciences, vol 7)

10. Buzsáki G, Ponomareff G, Bayardo F, Shaw T, Gage FH (1988) Suppression and induction of epileptic activity by neuronal grafts. Proc Natl Acad Sci USA 85: 9327–9330

11. Camu W, Marlier L, Lerner-Natoli M, Rondouin G, Privat A (1990) Transplantation of serotonergic neurons into the 5,7-DHT-lesioned rat olfactory bulb restores the parameters of kindling. Brain Res 815: 23–30

12. Chauvel P, Trottier S (1986) Role of noradrenergic ascending system in extinction of epileptic phenomena. Adv Neurol 44: 475–487

13. Clough RW, Browning RA, Maring ML, Jobe PC (1991) Intracerebral grafting of fetal dorsal pons in genetically epilepsy-prone rats: effects on audiogenic-induced seizures. Exp Neurol 112: 195–199

14. Daszuta A, Strecker RE, Brundin P, Björklund A (1989) Serotonin neurons grafted to the adult rat hippocampus: I. Time course of growth as studied by immunohistochemistry and biochemistry. Brain Res 458: 1–19

15. Daszuta A, Kalen P, Strecker RE, Brundin P, Björklund A (1989) Serotonin neurons grafted to the adult rat hippocampus. II. 5-HT release as studied by intracerebral microdialysis. Brain Res 498: 323–332

16. Emson PC, Joseph MH (1975) Neurochemical and morphological changes during the development of cobalt-induced epilepsy in the rat. Brain Res 93: 91–110

17. Fine A, Meldrum BS, Patel S (1990) Modulation of experimentally induced epilepsy by intracerebral grafts of fetal GABAergic neurons. Neuropsychologia 28: 627–634

18. Foote SL, Bloom FE, Aston-Jones G (1983) Nucleus locus coeruleus: new evidence of anatomical and physiological specificity. Physiol Rev 63: 844–911

19. Freedman R, Taylor DA, Seiger Å, Olson L, Hoffer BJ (1979) Seizures and related epileptiform activity in hippocampus transplanted to the anterior chamber of the eye: modulation by cholinergic and adrenergic input. Ann Neurol 6: 281–295

20. Gastaut H, Gastaut JL, Goncalves E, Silva GF, Fernandez Sanchez GR (1975) Relative frequency of different types of epilepsy: a study employing the classification of the International League Against Epilepsy. Epilepsia 16: 457–461

21. Gellman RL, Kallianos JA, McNamara JO (1987) Alpha-2 receptors mediate an endogenous noradrenergic suppression of kindling development. J Pharmacol Exp Ther 241: 891–898

22. Hoffer BJ, Seiger Å, Taylor D, Olson L, Freedman R (1977) Seizures and related epileptiform activity in hippocampus transplanted to the anterior chamber of the eye: I. Characterization of seizures, interictal spikes and synchronous activity. Exp Neurol 54: 233–250

23. Iadarola MJ, Gale K (1982) Substantia nigra: site of anticonvulsant activity mediated by γ-aminobutyric acid. Science 218: 1237–1240

24. Jimenez-Rivera CA, Weiss GK (1989) The effect of amygdala kindled seizures on locus coeruleus activity. Brain Res Bull 22: 751–758

25. Jobe PC, Laird HE, Ko K, Ray T, Daily JW (1982) Abnormalities in monoamine levels in the central nervous system of the genetically epilepsy-prone rat. Epilepsia 23: 359–366

26. Kamphuis W, Huisman E, Wadman WJ, Lopes da Silva FH (1989) Decrease in GABA immunoreactivity and alteration of GABA metabolism after kindling in the rat hippocampus. Exp Brain Res 74: 375–386

27. Kamphuis W, Wadman WJ, Buijs RM, Lopes da Silva FH (1986) Decrease in number of hippocampal gamma-aminobutyric acid (GABA) immunoreactive cells in the rat kindling model of epilepsy. Exp Brain Res 64: 491–495

28. Laird HE, II, Dailey JW, Jobe PC (1984) Neurotransmitter abnormalities in genetically epileptic rodents. Fed Proc 43: 2505–2509

29. Lauterborn JC, Ribak CE (1989) Differences in dopamine beta-hydroxylase immunoreactivity between the brains of genetically epilepsy-prone and Sprague-Dawley rats. Epilepsy Res 4: 161–176

30. Lerner-Natoli M, Rondouin G, Malafosse A, Sandillon F, Privat A, Baldy-Moulinier M (1986) Facilitation of olfactory bulb kindling after specific destruction of serotoninergic terminals in the olfactory bulb of the rat. Neurosci Lett 66: 299–304

31. Lindvall O, Bengzon J, Brundin P, Kalén P, Kokaia M (1990) Locus coeruleus grafts in hippocampal kindling epilepsy: noradrenaline release, receptor specificity and influence on seizure development. Prog Brain Res 82: 339–346

32. McIntyre DC, Racine RJ (1986) Kindling mechanisms: current progress of an experimental epilepsy model. Prog Neurobiol 27: 1–12

33. McNamara JO (1984) Kindling: an animal model of complex partial epilepsy. Ann Neurol 16 [Suppl]: S72–S76

34. McNamara JO, Galloway MT, Rigsbee LC, Shin C (1984) Evidence implicating substantia nigra in regulation of kindled seizure threshold. Neuroscience 4: 2410–2417
35. Murata Y, Chiba T, Brundin P, Björklund A, Lindvall O (1990) Formation of synaptic graft-host connections by noradrenergic locus coeruleus neurons transplanted into the adult rat hippocampus. Exp Neurol 110: 258–267
36. Olson L, Freedman R, Seiger Å, Hoffer B (1977) Electrophysiology and cytology of hippocampal formation transplants in the anterior chamber of the eye: 1. Intrinsic organization. Brain Res 119: 87–106
37. Olson L, Seiger Å, Hoffer BJ, Taylor D (1979) Isolated catecholaminergic projections from substantia nigra and locus coeruleus to caudate, hippocampus and cerebral cortex formed by intraocular sequential double brain grafts. Exp Brain Res 35: 47–67
38. Olson L, Seiger Å, Taylor D, Freedman R, Hoffer BJ (1980) Conditions for adrenergic hyperinnervation in hippocampus: I. Histochemical evidence from intraocular double grafts. Exp Brain Res 39: 277–288
39. Piredda S, Gale K (1985) A crucial epileptogenic site in deep prepyriform cortex. Nature 317: 623–625
40. Racine RJ (1972) Modification of seizure activity by electrical stimulation: II. Motor seizure. Electroencephalogr Clin Neurophysiol 32: 284–294
41. Racine RJ, Burnham WM (1984) The kindling model. In: Schwartzkroin PA, Wheal HV (eds) Electrophysiology of epilepsy. Academic, London, pp 153–171
42. Ribak CE, Harris AB, Vaughn JE, Roberts E (1979) Inhibitory, GABAergic nerve terminals decrease at sites of focal epilepsy. Science 205: 211–214
43. Schwartzkroin PA, Kunkel DD (1988) Viability of GABAergic striatal neurons grafted into normal hippocampus. Soc Neurosci Abstr 233.8.
44. Sirinathsinghji DJS, Dunnett SB, Isacson O, Clarke DJ, Kendrick K, Björklund A (1988) Striatal grafts in rats with unilateral neostriatal lesions: II. In vivo monitoring of GABA release in globus pallidus and substantia nigra. Neuroscience 24: 803–811
45. Stevens JR, Phillips I, de Beaurepaire R (1988) Gamma-vinyl GABA in endopiriform area suppresses kindled amygdala seizures. Epilepsia 29: 404–411
46. Stevens JR, Phillips I, Freed WJ, Poltorak M (1988) Cerebral transplants for seizures: preliminary results. Epilepsia 29: 731–737
47. Taylor D, Freedman R, Seiger Å, Olson L, Hoffer BJ (1980) Conditions for adrenergic hyperinnervation in hippocampus: II. Electrophysiological evidence from intraocular double grafts. Exp Brain Res 39: 289–299
48. Wada JA, Sato M, Corcoran ME (1974) Persistent seizure susceptibility and recurrent spontaneous seizures in kindled cats. Epilepsia 15: 465–478
49. Wictorin K, Björklund A (1989) Connectivity of striatal grafts implanted into the ibotenic acid-lesioned striatum: II. Cortical afferents. Neuroscience 30: 297–311
50. Wictorin K, Isacson O, Fischer W, Nothias F, Peschanski M, Björklund A (1988) Connectivity of striatal grafts implanted into the ibotenic acid-lesioned striatum: I. Subcortical afferents. Neuroscience 27: 547–562
51. Wictorin K, Simerly RB, Isacson O, Swanson LW, Björklund A. (1989) Connectivity of striatal grafts implanted into the ibotenic acid-lesioned striatum: III. Efferent projecting graft neurons and their relation to host afferents within the grafts. Neuroscience 30: 313–330

Genetically Modified Cells for Intracerebral Transplantation

F. H. Gage and L. J. Fisher

Department of Neurosciences, Clinical Sciences Building, University of California, San Diego, La Jolla, California, USA

Introduction

Cells have been implanted into the central nervous system (CNS) since the end of the last century [61]. However, only within the past two decades has intracerebral grafting (ICG) become a viable technique for exploring the functioning of the CNS and repairing damaged neural structures [23]. In most studies to date, embryonic neural tissues have been used as donor material for ICG, since these cells survive well within the CNS and effectively replace damaged or missing neural components.

While neural cells have been found to provide potent functional restoration in some animal models of CNS disorders (see the chapters by Bengzon and Lindvall, Björklund and Wictorin, Brundin and Lindvall, and Dunnett in this volume), the extension of neural grafting into the clinical domain poses several problems. In particular, the necessity of using fetal tissue as donor material has clear ethical ramifications, and there are concerns over achieving successful immunologic incorporation of the donor tissue into the host environment (see the chapter by Widner in this volume). For these and other reasons, many investigators have explored the use of nonneural cells, such as glia or adrenal medulla cells, as alternative donor materials for ICG.

If such cells are initially obtained from the host candidate, problems with immunologic rejection may be virtually eliminated. However, there are several factors to consider when using any host-derived nonneural cells for ICG. First, the part of the body from which cells are obtained must be able to function effectively once the cells are removed. Second, the donor cells must be able to survive in the new location, and, third, the donor cells must synthesize and secrete a molecule of interest in quantities that are sufficient to replace or restore normal CNS functioning. Still, cells selected according to such criteria may not always prove optimal for ICG; in many instances, it has been difficult to obtain robust survival and functioning of nonneural cells within the CNS unless they were derived from embryonic or very young donors.

Since it is now possible to introduce new genetic material efficiently into the genome of cells, it is no longer necessary to restrict potential donor-cell candidates for ICG to those that normally produce a given desired substance. The strategy of using genetically modified cells for ICG was first described by Gage and colleagues in 1987 [25] and has subsequently developed into a viable technique for the site-specific delivery of discrete molecules to the brain. This chapter will discuss the gene transfer/ICG technique and describe some of the uses of genetically modified cells for correcting a regional deficit in the brain. While there are overlapping issues related to the concept of "gene therapy" in general, this chapter will focus on the interface between gene therapy and neuroscience.

There are a variety of reasons to modify a cell genetically, including (1) to investigate the function of a gene and its product, (2) to study regulatory elements related to a gene and its product, (3) to mark cells at a particular time for lineage analyses, (4) to kill a selected population of cells, (5) to transform cells into an immortalized or conditionally immortalized cell line, (6) to correct a defective gene in a host cell, (7) to use the modified cells to secrete a product that could correct a deficit in a target organ, and (8) to create transgenic animals. The notion of correcting a defective gene in a host cell or, more broadly, to correct a disease phenotype in whole animals has been termed somatic gene therapy [22]. Such therapy would be accomplished either by modification of the expression of a resident mutant gene or through the introduction of new genetic information into defective cells or organs in vivo. For neurologic dysfunctions, a somatic gene therapy approach would require the development of effective vectors for delivering foreign genetic sequences ("transgenes") to neurons or other cells within the CNS. Since techniques for achieving somatic gene therapy through site-specific correction or replacement of gene sequences are not yet well developed, most current models of gene therapy rely on techniques of genetic augmentation rather than replacement.

In a diseased organism, an alternative to somatic gene therapy would be to modify individual cells genetically in vitro and then to graft them into the host in order for them to provide deficient molecules in vivo. This approach has been pursued for several years for systemic disorders and was recently used in the treatment of adenosine deaminase deficiency [17], an immunodeficiency disease that is fatal in the absence of a therapeutic intervention. Similarly, the ICG of genetically modified cells may prove to be a powerful treatment for some CNS disorders. The strategy for grafting ge-

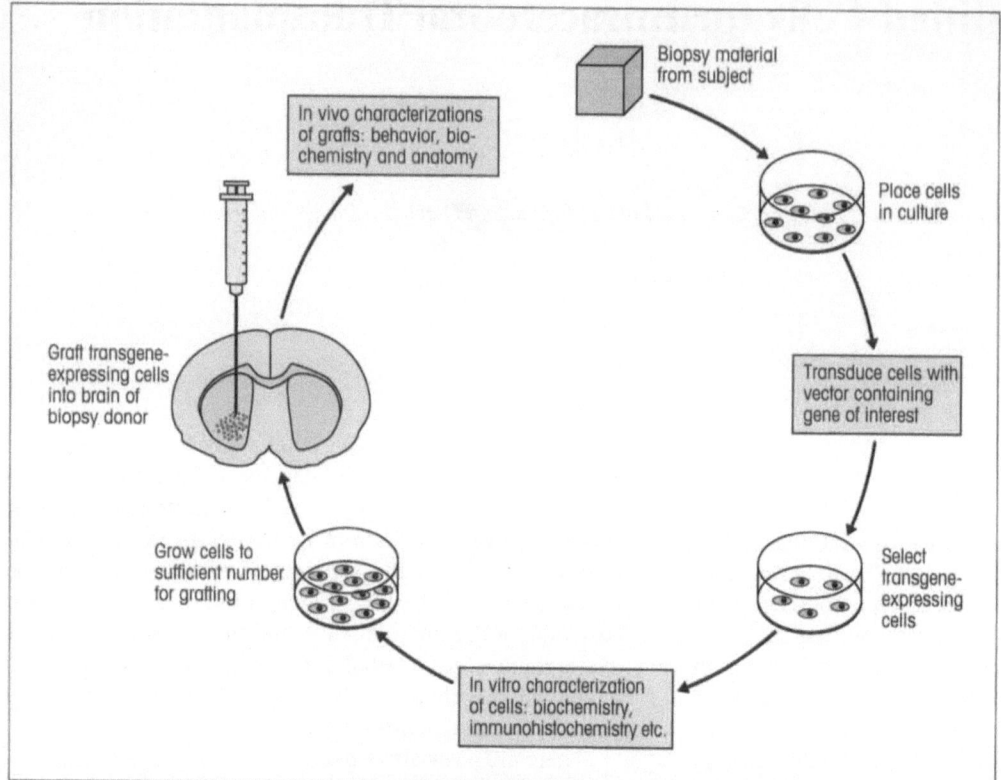

Fig. 1. *Schematic illustration of the gene transfer/ICG strategy. To minimize adverse immune responses, donor cells are obtained from the future graft recipient for genetic modification and ICG. The gene of interest is inserted into the cells in vitro by means of one of a variety of gene transfer techniques. The cells that successfully express the transgene are characterized in vitro and then grown to sufficient quantities for grafting. The original donor of the cells receives one or more deposits of the genetically modified cells in discrete areas of the brain. At various intervals after grafting, the survival and functioning of the implanted cells is assessed*

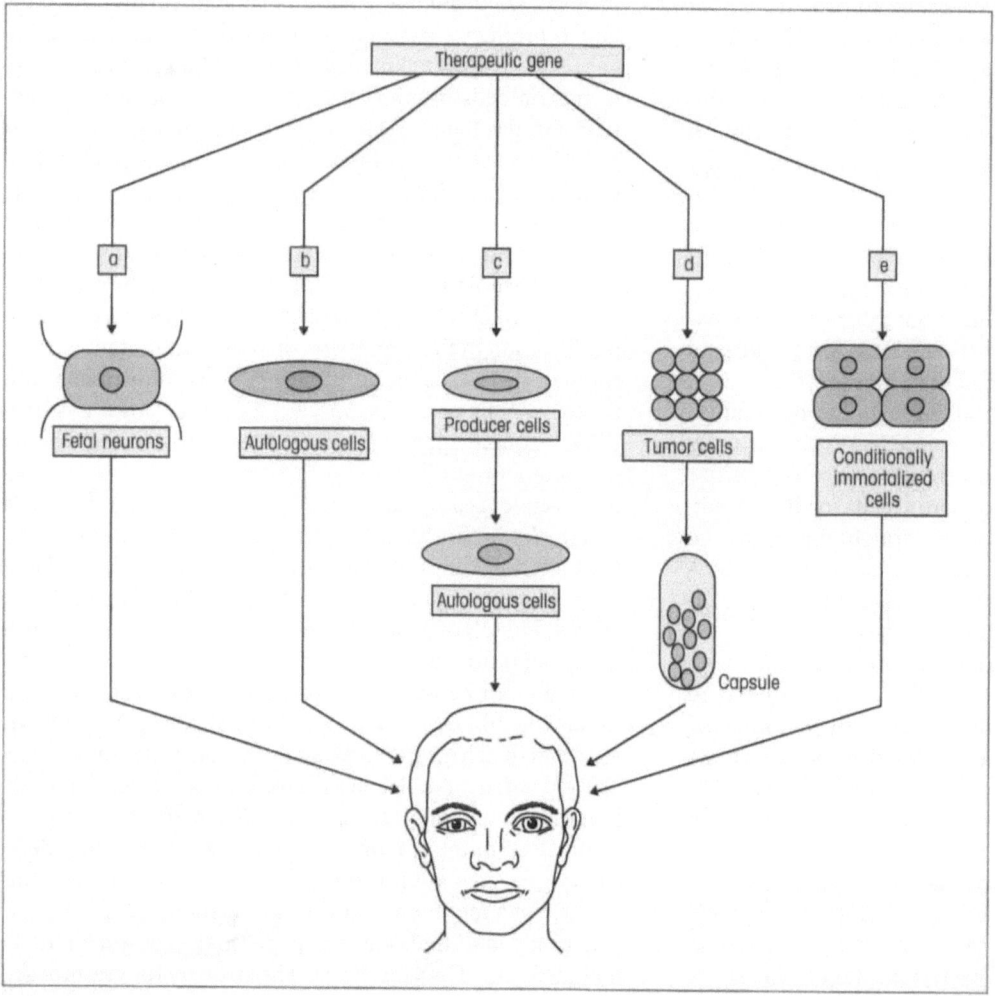

Fig. 2. *Schematic illustration of different cell populations that may be useful for genetic modification and ICG. A therapeutic gene is shown being inserted into five potential cellular recipients (a–e). Fetal neurons (a) would probably achieve the best graft-host interaction but do not currently survive well through culturing, gene transfer, and ICG procedures. Further, fetal cells may elicit adverse immunologic responses after ICG. Cells obtained from the future graft recipient (autologous cells) would evoke the least immunologic reactions after ICG; such cells, which must be mitotic, may be genetically modified by either transfection (b) or retroviral infection (c) (mediated through "producer cells") techniques. Tumor cells (d) are most amenable to gene transfer techniques, since they grow very well in culture. However, such growth would be detrimental in vivo and would need to be restricted either through encapsulation (**capsule**) or through antimitotic treatment prior to grafting. Alternatively, immortalized cells (e) may be transfected to express a gene that will limit growth under physiologic conditions (conditionally immortalized cells)*

Fig. 3. Schematic illustration of two common methods of gene transfer. In the retroviral infection technique (**upper left**), retroviral particles are used as carriers of RNA fragments containing the gene of interest (transgene, **shaded region**). These particles bind to receptors on donor cells and release their RNA cargo into the cell cytoplasm. There, the RNA is converted into DNA that is then incorporated into the host genome. Once incorporated, the new gene directs the production of new proteins (transgene proteins). Another gene transfer technique is the lipofection method (**bottom right**). In this method, DNA containing the gene of interest (**darkened region**) is mixed in a solution with charged lipid particles to form a DNA-liposome complex. These positively charged complexes bind to the negatively charged cellular membrane and release the DNA into the cytoplasm. The DNA is then incorporated into the host DNA and directs the synthesis of new proteins

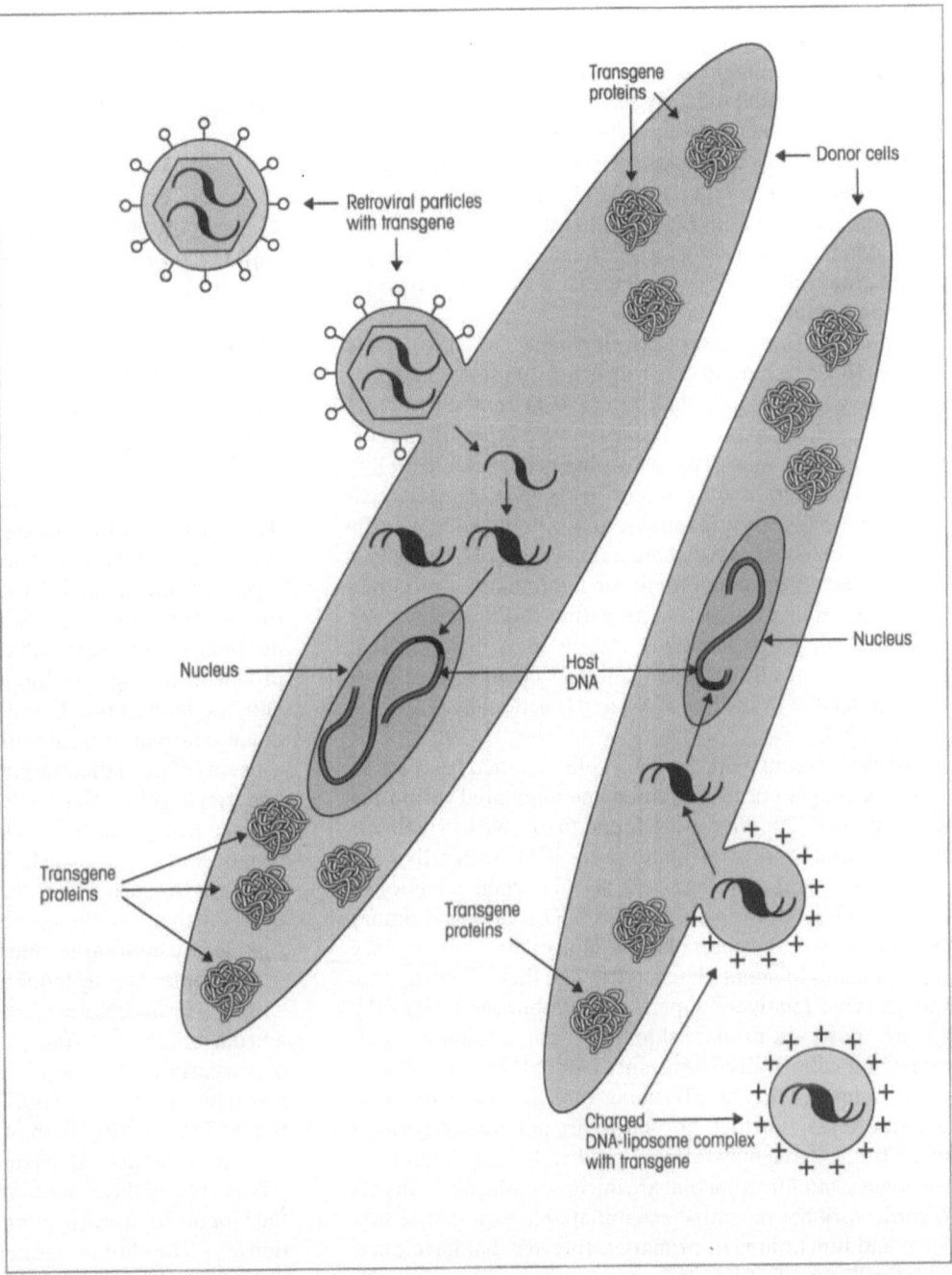

netically altered cells into the brain includes the following basic steps (Fig. 1): (1) select and prepare donor cells from a primary biopsy or from established cell lines, (2) transfer the gene of interest into the cultured donor cells, (3) select the cells that express the transgene and/or synthesize the transgene product at a desired level in vitro, (4) graft the modified cells into the brain of the biopsy donor, and (5) assess graft survival and function in vivo.

In general, the criteria used to select a cell for genetic modification and ICG differ little from those used to select any other cell type for ICG. The cells should elicit minimal immune responses from the host, survive in a stable state within the CNS, and show sustained production of the substance(s) of interest. However, there are additional factors to consider when selecting cells for genetic modification, e.g., the ability of the cells to survive well in vitro and to exhibit sustained proliferation during the gene transfer procedures.

There are a variety of replicating host-derived cells that may be appropriate for genetic modification and ICG, e.g., bone marrow cells, skin fibroblasts, endothelial cells, and hepatocytes (Fig. 2). Such cells, though, are solely secretory and would be unable to establish functional interconnections with host tissues. A graft containing genetically modified peripheral cells may function as either an autonomous biologic pump of a given substance or a receptacle for metabolizing and/or eliminating toxic compounds from the brain. To achieve the synaptic incorporation of grafted cells into the host environment, it may be necessary to consider the use of neurons for genetic modification. However, primary neurons maintained for prolonged periods in culture have not been found to survive well after ICG [9, 47]. While certain neuronal cell lines have been reported to persist for prolonged periods in culture [53], they will be foreign to most hosts and may retain undesirable growth characteristics after implantation. Further, it is unclear whether the connections formed by genetically modified neurons implanted into ectopic locations of the CNS would be functionally meaningful.

Through the early development of the gene transfer/ICG technique, most investigators selected donor cells for genetic manipulation and ICG that showed favorable in vitro characteristics: they were typically immortalized cell lines that were easily obtained, survived well in culture, and were readily amenable to gene transfer techniques. Perhaps not surprisingly, such cells did not generally display favorable in vivo characteristics after ICG: specifically, in the absence of antimitotic treatment the modified cell lines often formed tumors within the brain [37, 62]. Nonetheless, several studies clearly demonstrated that grafts of genetically modified cell lines could restore deficient molecules in the brain [38] and functionally affect the host [37, 67].

In more recent work, primary cells obtained from a skin biopsy were genetically modified and implanted within the donor animal [20]. They were found to survive in a well-delineated area for several months after ICG. Such cells were also shown to effectively reverse the abnormal behavior of the hosts [20]. For the gene transfer/ICG approach, primary fibroblasts have the particular advantages that they are easy to obtain and to manipulate in vitro and that, as autografts, they survive relatively unperturbed within the brain [41]. Clearly, however, primary skin fibroblasts will not be optimal donor cells in all circumstances, since they naturally secrete molecules that may be undesirable in a particular system of interest. Further, fibroblasts are not normally found in the brain, and it may be more prudent to seek donor cells for genetic modification that are intrinsic to the CNS. In this regard, work has recently been initiated to explore the survival and functioning of primary astrocytes that have been genetically modified [39, 45].

Once a cell type has been selected for genetic modification, there are a variety of gene transfer techniques for inserting a gene of interest into these cells (Fig. 3). Such techniques were developed to enhance the efficiency with which DNA penetrates cells and incorporates into the host genome. Perhaps one of the most common techniques is the retroviral infection method, which achieves rapid gene transfer into a wide variety of donor cells. One potential limitation of the retroviral method, though, is that the size of the DNA for the gene of interest that can be carried by the virus is restricted. To date, the two most frequently utilized transgenes in ICG experiments – namely tyrosine hydroxylase, the biosynthetic enzyme in the catecholamine pathway, and nerve growth factor (NGF), a molecule with trophic effects on the cholinergic system – have been delivered into donor cells by means of both retroviral and other gene transfer methods. At present, the type of technique used for gene transfer does not appear to influence the level of expression of the gene after its insertion.

Genetically Modified Cells and the Neurotrophic Strategy

Many disorders of the CNS are characterized by the progressive deterioration or dysfunction of neurons and a subsequent loss of neurochemical communication between cells. One of the potential therapeutic uses for genetically modified cells may be to supply neurotrophic agents to diseased neurons and intervene in a degenerative process. Evidence from a variety of conditions indicates that neuronal survival in vivo may depend on the presence of an adequate supply of neurotrophic factors. The concept is supported by the existence of such phenomena as (1) "developmental neuronal death," in which the excessive number of neurons produced during development is decreased to accommodate the limited number of target cells [15, 33]; (2) "retrograde neuronal degeneration," in which axotomized neurons cut off from their target cells and surrounding glial cells undergo degeneration or death [16, 29, 51]; and (3) "pathologic neuronal death," in which specific populations of neurons degenerate and die [3, 65]. One explanation commonly put forth for such occurrences is that neurons normally depend for their continued health upon neurotrophic factors supplied by their target and associated glial cells; disruption in this trophic supply induces cellular death.

The cholinergic projection from the adult rat septum and diagonal band to the ipsilateral hippocampus has been a particularly useful model for examining the role of neurotrophic agents within the CNS. Neurons of the medial septum and the vertical limb of the diagonal band project dorsally to the hippocampus through the fimbria-fornix [4, 24]. About 50% of these neurons are cholinergic [1] and provide the hippocampus with about 90% of its cholinergic innervation [59]. The cholinergic neurons, axons, and terminals can be visualized by histochemical localization of acetylcholinesterase (AChE) [10, 55] and choline acetyltransferase (ChAT) [4, 55], and the terminal fields within the hippocampal formation can be quantified biochemically by measuring the extracted ChAT activity [21].

Complete transection of the fimbria-fornix pathway in adult rats results in the rapid and complete retrograde degeneration and death of both cholinergic and noncholinergic neurons within the septum and diagonal band area [27, 34, 66]. One explanation for this axotomy-induced cell death is that the septal neurons become deprived of a critical supply of neurotrophic factors that may be provided by the postsynaptic neurons or glial cells in the axonal and/or synaptic vicinity of the hippocampal innervation territory [7, 13, 26, 50]. That this hippocampal factor may be NGF or an NGF-like substance is supported by studies showing that

Fig. 4. *Schematic illustration of the neurotrophic delivery strategy in the septal-hippocampal system. Sagittal sections through the brain show neurons within the septum/diagonal band extending axons through the fimbria to the hippocampus* (**top**). *The* **middle section** *shows the loss and degeneration of neurons within the septal region following the removal of the fimbria-fornix pathway. In the* **bottom figure**, *NGF-producing cells implanted into the septum (dark shapes within the upper portion of the septal area) deliver trophic support to damaged neurons (NGF diffuses throughout the septal area) and induce the regeneration of cholinergic processes*

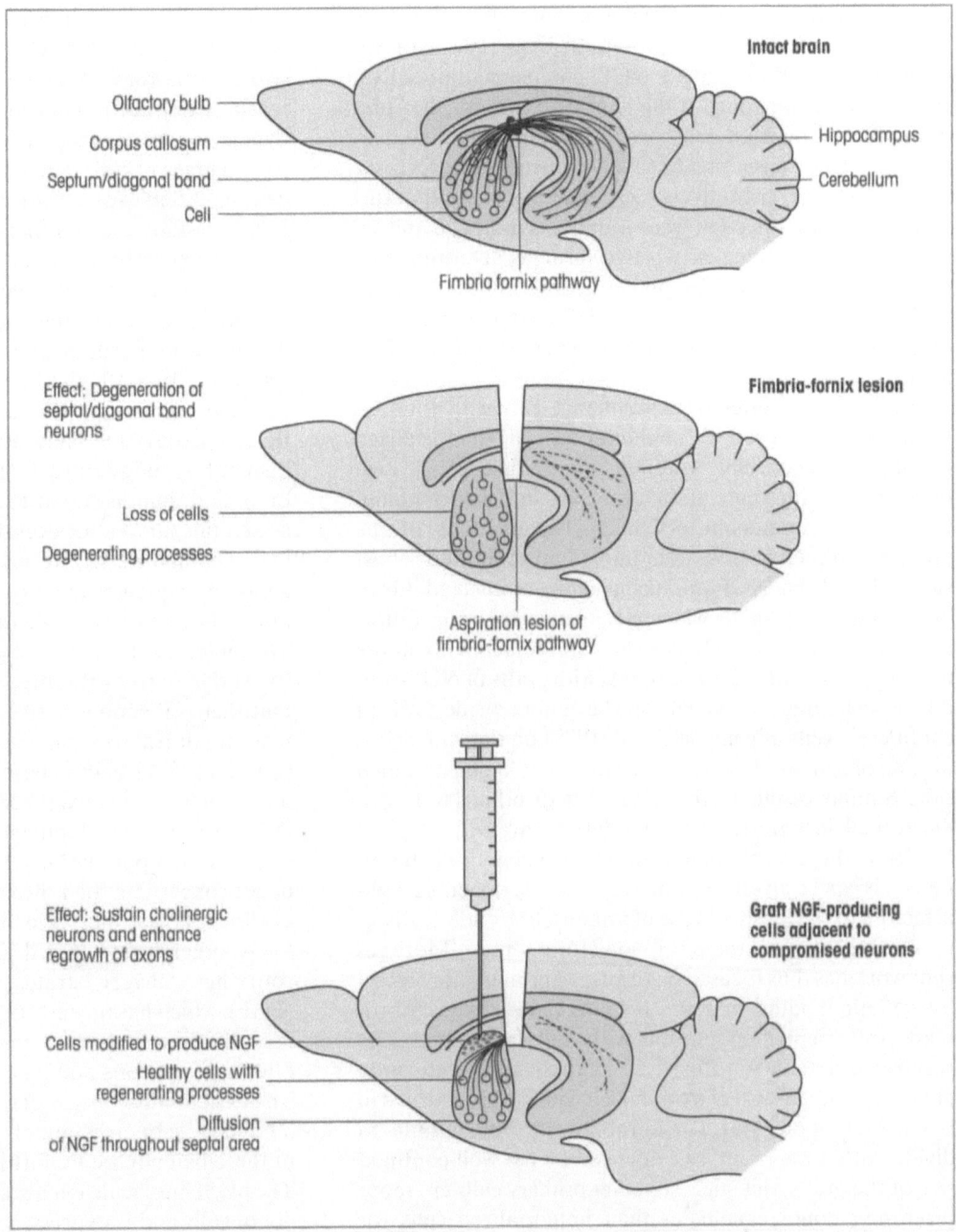

NGF levels within the brain are highest within target areas of the cholinoceptive basal forebrain systems.

NGF is the best characterized of the currently identified neurotrophic factors [5, 31, 60]. NGF supports the survival and axon growth of both sensory and sympathetic neurons in vitro and in vivo [11, 32]; NGF also attracts and guides regenerating axons [32] and may stimulate the axon growth rate even of neurons that do not require NGF for survival [14]. In the cholinergic system, radiolabeled NGF has been found to be transported retrogradely to the cell bodies of cholinergic neurons in the nucleus basalis after its injection into cortical target fields [57, 58]. Further, NGF administration has been found to increase ChAT activity in neuronal cultures [35, 36, 46, 48] and within the hippocampus and striatum of the rat brain [48].

Several groups [34, 66] have independently reported that the intracerebroventricular administration of purified NGF into adult rat brain from the time of the fimbria-fornix transection onwards prevents the death of most of the axotomized cholinergic neurons of the septal/diagonal band area. NGF administration also seems to prevent the degeneration of the cut septal cholinergic axons and/or to stimulate their regrowth, since a large number of AChE-positive cholinergic fibers appear to form a neuroma-like structure proximal to the transection site [27].

In this model, therefore, secretory cells genetically modified to produce NGF may prove particularly effective in providing site-specific delivery of neurotrophic support to delay or halt the degeneration of axotomized cholinergic neurons (Fig. 4). This possibility was explored initially by using immortalized fibroblasts as donor cells for genetic manipulation and ICG. A prototypical retroviral vector was constructed that contained NGF complementary DNA (cDNA) corresponding to the shorter transcript that predominates in mouse tissue receiving sympathetic innervation [18]. This transcript is believed to encode the precursor to NGF that is constitutively secreted. Fibroblasts that survived retroviral infection were found to synthesize and secrete NGF in a biologically active form, as determined by the ability of the NGF to induce neurite outgrowth from PC12 rat pheochromocytoma cells [30]. Noninfected fibroblasts do not normally produce detectable levels of NGF in vitro.

In an initial series of experiments, rats with fimbria-fornix lesions received implantations of immortalized fibroblasts genetically modified to produce NGF [54]. Control rats with similar lesions received implants of noninfected cells. Immunohistochemical examinations of the grafts performed 2 weeks after implantation showed robust survival of both NGF-producing and noninfected fibroblasts. However, there was a clear between-group difference in the number of cholinergic neurons surviving in the medial septum: whereas in animals with grafts of NGF-producing cells there remained on the lesioned side 92% of cholinergic cells as compared with 100% on the intact side, in control animals there remained only 49% on the lesioned side. Similar results were obtained with other NGF-producing cell lines grafted in this model system [19].

While these results demonstrated that genetically modified cells can be an effective delivery vehicle of neurotrophic factors to the brain, the use of immortalized cells for ICG is not optimal, since these cells may form tumors. More recent work has thus focused on the use of primary fibroblasts for genetic modification and ICG. In these studies, fibroblast grafts implanted into rats with fimbria-fornix lesions survived in a stable state for several months and significantly enhanced the survival of axotomized cholinergic neurons in the medial septum [43]. The fibroblasts did not continue to divide within the brain, as evidenced by the well-confined size of the grafts; this suggested that primary cells are more promising donor candidates than immortalized cells for achieving the long-term survival and functioning of genetically modified cells transplanted into the brain.

The cellular delivery of neurotrophic agents to the brain may also be an effective method for delaying the degenerative loss of neurons that occurs during aging. Several laboratories have demonstrated that shrinkage and loss of cholinergic neurons take place in the basal forebrain of aged animals and humans [6, 65], changes that appear to be correlated with a decrease in cognitive ability [16]. While it is clear that several systems undergo degenerative changes in aging, the age-related changes in cholinergic neurons provide a good model for neurotrophic delivery by grafts of genetically modified cells. In preliminary work, NGF-producing fibroblasts were implanted into the nucleus basalis of aged rats and their effect on learning and memory assessed; aged-matched control animals received noninfected fibroblasts instead [12]. The aged animals with NGF-producing grafts performed significantly better than the controls in a water maze task. These observations and those made in rats with fimbria-fornix lesions provide strong evidence that the localized application of exogenous neurotrophic support to damaged neurons may delay the progression of degenerative changes in cells. Secretory cells that have been genetically modified to produce essential neurotrophic factors can be successfully used for that purpose.

The neurotrophic strategy using genetically modified cells will certainly grow to encompass a variety of additional molecules. Several other neurotrophic factors have been isolated and purified and their cDNAs cloned and sequenced. Two of these molecules, brain-derived neurotrophic factor (BDNF) and neurotrophin 3 (NT-3), are thought to be of the same family as NGF, as suggested by sequence homology and activity. BDNF was isolated from pig brain and demonstrated to be active in an assay that assessed the survival of dorsal root ganglia neurons in vitro [44]. The mature BDNF and NGF proteins share four regions of sequence identity, comprising over 70% of the molecules, and have four regions of divergent sequences. The biologic actions of recombinant NT-3 have been shown to overlap partly with those of NGF and BDNF, to the extent that NT-3 induces fiber outgrowth from sympathetic neurons, dorsal root ganglia, nodose ganglion sensory neurons, and PC12 cells. These observations suggest that the neurotrophins may exert combinatorial or sequential regulation over the development and differentiation of responsive neuronal populations. To date, there is no in vivo evidence concerning the range or nature of the trophic effects of either of these factors in the CNS.

Another factor that deserves consideration in a neurotrophic delivery strategy is fibroblast growth factor (FGF), which has recently been established as a protein that is synthesized in the nervous system and exerts a variety of effects on neurons and glia, both in vivo and in vitro [28]. The FGF family consists of seven members that share about 30%–60% sequence homology, with the best characterized of these being basic FGF (bFGF) and acidic FGF (aFGF). The bFGF molecule is a heparin-binding mitogen for a variety of cells and is expressed in several types of neuroectodermal cells. There have been several reports that bFGF has trophic effects on cholinergic neurons in vivo [2] and cortical and hippocampal neurons in vitro [49, 64]. In general, bFGF has been shown to have both neurotrophic (affecting cell survival) and neurotropic (affecting the direction of axon growth) activities; it is therefore not considered a "classic" trophic factor. However, its action in CNS wound healing certainly indicates that it may be a broadly active neurotrophic factor of potential therapeutic use in neurodegenerative diseases.

Genetically Modified Cells for Neurotransmitter Replacement

The loss of neurons in neurodegenerative disorders ultimately results in a substantial decline in neurotransmitter

Fig. 5. Schematic illustration of the rotational paradigm. Shown are coronal sections of the rat brain at the level of the striatum. The **left-hand drawings** show dopamine receptor numbers, and the **right-hand drawings** show dopamine levels. In the intact brain (**top sections**), the striatum has relatively equal numbers of dopamine receptors and dopamine levels in the two hemispheres. After the unilateral destruction by 6-hydroxydopamine of dopaminergic inputs from the substantia nigra to the striatum, there is in the denervated striatum an increase in dopamine receptors and a loss of dopamine levels (**middle sections**). Drugs that interact with the dopaminergic system cause abnormal behavior in these animals. For example, the dopamine-receptor-stimulating drug apomorphine (**left bottom section**) strongly activates the denervated striatum and evokes a walking pattern away from the side of the lesion (a lesion in the left hemisphere elicits clockwise rotation). Conversely, the dopamine-releasing drug amphetamine stimulates dopamine release predominantly from the intact striatum (**right bottom section**) and thus elicits a circular walking pattern towards the side of the lesion (a lesion in the left hemisphere elicits counterclockwise rotation)

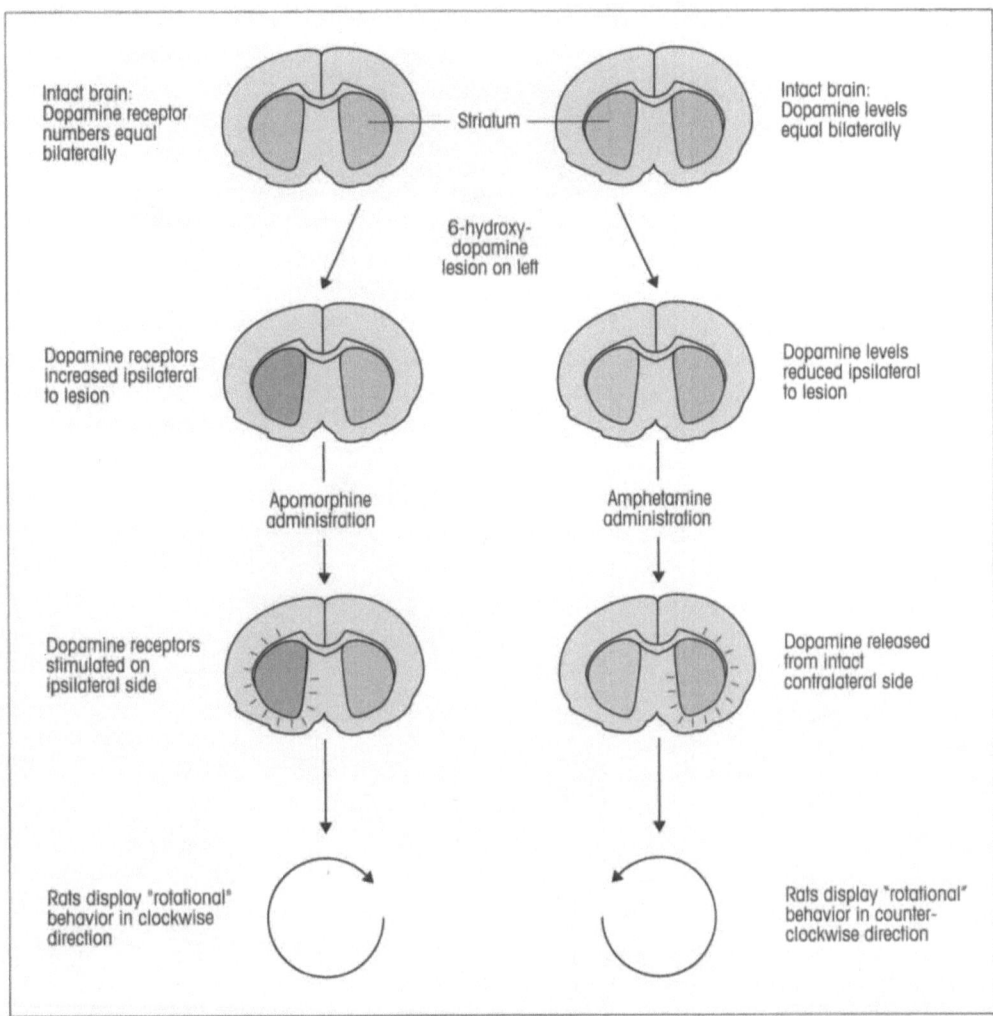

levels and an impairment of neural processing. Consequently, therapeutic interventions for many CNS diseases have focused on the systemic oral administration of neurotransmitter precursors in an attempt to elevate the levels of depleted transmitters within the brain. The extent and nature of the transmitter loss, however, clearly influence the effectiveness of such interventions. For example, Alzheimer's disease (AD) is characterized by a substantial loss or disruption of both cholinergic and noncholinergic systems within the brain [40]. However, to date most pharmacologic treatments of AD have focused on the supplementation of cholinergic function alone [6]. These targeted treatments have generally met with limited success. Conversely, Parkinson's disease is characterized predominantly by a loss of the pigmented dopaminergic neurons of the substantia nigra, pars compacta. In this disease, the systemic administration of L-dopa, the precursor of dopamine, has proved to be a very effective treatment of the motor impairments.

There is an animal model of Parkinson's disease in which lesions are created by the local intracerebral administration of the catecholamine neurotoxin 6-hydroxydopamine. Rats with unilateral lesions show a spontaneous postural bias towards the side of the lesion and walk in a circle (rotate) after

the systemic injection of a dopamine agonist [63] (Fig. 5). These behaviors do not have particular clinical relevance, but they do reflect the dopamine imbalance in the animal's brain and provide a model for exploring the effectiveness of dopamine replacement (Fig. 6).

A substantial amount of literature demonstrates that the ICG of fetal dopaminergic neurons into rats with lesions caused by 6-hydroxydopamine induces significant improvement of motor, sensory, and cognitive abnormalities. The results have been so promising that hundreds of parkinsonian patients have received intracerebral implants of adrenal or fetal dopaminergic tissue (see the chapter by Brundin and Lindvall in this volume). Although the clinical results have been somewhat inconclusive, the strategy of inserting a source of dopamine directly into affected areas of the brain appears to be valid. Therefore, in Parkinson's disease genetically modified cells may be a particularly suitable method for supplementing dopamine levels, since immunologic problems may be avoided by using cells from the patient for genetic modification.

A number of studies have examined the survival and functioning of genetically modified cells implanted into rats with lesions caused by 6-hydroxydopamine. In this model

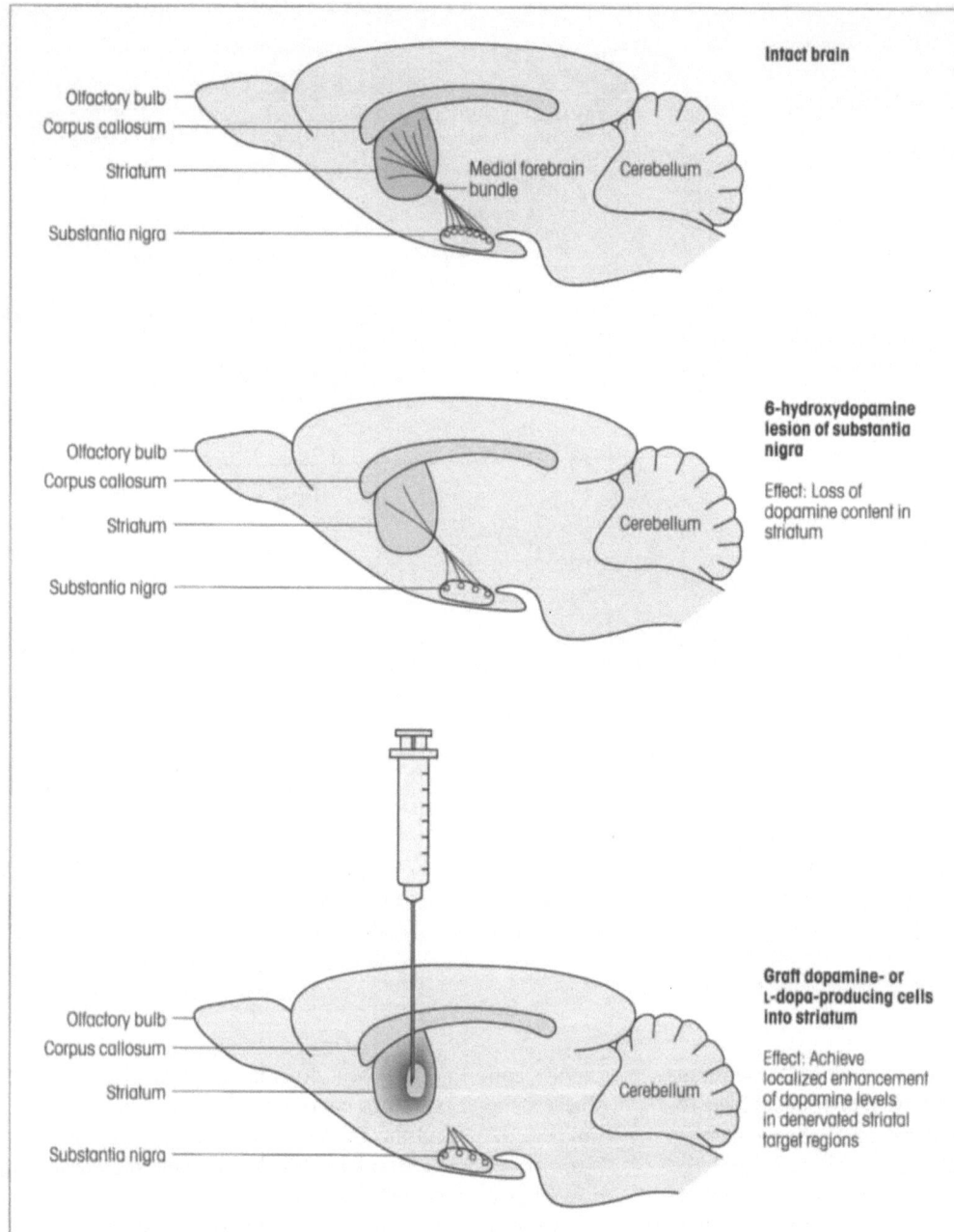

Fig. 6. *Schematic illustration of the neurotransmitter replacement strategy in the nigrostriatal system. Sagittal sections through the brain show the dopaminergic neurons within the pars compacta of the substantia nigra projecting to the striatum through the medial forebrain bundle. Green color (**top**) represents normal levels of dopamine within the striatum. In the **middle drawing**, most of the dopaminergic neurons within the substantia nigra have been removed by the intracerebral infusion of 6-hydroxydopamine, with resulting substantial reduction of dopamine content in the striatum (**light green**). In the **bottom drawing**, cells producing dopamine or l-dopa are shown implanted in the striatum. These cells induce a localized increase in dopamine levels within the striatum (**darker green area around the graft**) and normalize functioning*

system, the transgene typically selected for study has been tyrosine hydroxylase (TH), the enzyme that converts tyrosine to L-dopa. Cells genetically altered to express TH will have the capacity to form L-dopa, but not dopamine, unless they endogenously contain dopa decarboxylase, the enzyme that catalyzes the conversion of L-dopa to dopamine.

In initial work, several groups introduced a TH transgene into immortalized cells. Cells expressing TH showed positive immunoreactivity for TH in vitro and readily synthesized and released L-dopa into the culture medium [37, 62, 67]. To assess the ability of the TH-expressing cells to continue to produce TH and secrete L-dopa in vivo, the modified cells were implanted into the striata of rats with lesions induced by 6-hydroxydopamine. Histologic exami-

nations performed 2 weeks after the ICG revealed cell survival [37, 62, 67] and the continued synthesis of TH protein [37, 62]. In vivo microdialysis of the host striata indicated that L-dopa was released from the grafts and rapidly converted to dopamine within the host brain [38]. Further, behavioral tests of the rats with implants showed a significant amelioration of drug-induced locomotor activity [37, 67]. However, it was clear from these studies that immortalized cells were not optimal for use in vivo, since they often continued to multiply after ICG [37, 38, 62].

More recent studies in the rat model of Parkinson's disease have explored the use of primary cells for genetic manipulation and ICG [20, 39, 45]. Fisher and colleagues used primary fibroblasts obtained from a skin biopsy as cellular recipients of a TH transgene [20]. These cells displayed TH activity and L-dopa production that were comparable to those seen previously in immortalized fibroblasts. The cells were implanted into rats with lesions induced by 6-hydroxydopamine, and the animals' behavior was assessed every 2 weeks for 8 weeks after grafting. The control animals also had lesions but received grafts of noninfected fibroblasts. The TH-expressing cells induced a marked decrease in abnormal locomotor activity 2 weeks after grafting that persisted for 8 weeks. However, the graft effect did diminish with time, which suggested a decreased in vivo functioning or survival of the cells during the 8-week observation period. (This hypothesis was consistent with the finding that intracerebral grafts of noninfected primary fibroblasts significantly decreased in volume between 1 and 3 weeks after grafting and then stabilized for up to 8 weeks [42].) Ten weeks after grafting, histochemical examination showed the presence of TH messenger RNA and TH protein only within the grafts containing TH-expressing fibroblasts.

Discussion and Future Directions

The ICG of genetically modified cells is a powerful method for achieving the site-specific delivery of a discrete compound to the CNS. In a clinical setting, such cells may provide a method for intervening in the degenerative loss of neurons or for supplementing substances that are depleted in the damaged brain. For therapeutic application, primary fibroblasts or other cells could be obtained from the patient, cultured in vitro, and transfected with a gene that is appropriate for the neurologic disorder to be treated by ICG. For example, tyrosine hydroxylase without or with dopa decarboxylase could be used for dopamine replacement in Parkinson's disease. Alternatively, combining both trophic factor and neurotransmitter delivery may be considered for disorders such as Alzheimer's disease, where it may be possible to delay neuronal cholinergic degeneration through NGF delivery and restore acetylcholine levels. Schinstine et al. recently reported that fibroblasts transfected with the gene for Drosophila choline acetyltransferase can produce and secrete biologically active acetylcholine [56]. Although these strategies would not cure the disorders, they might provide an approach for delaying their progression or reduce the severity of symptoms. Prior to any clinical use, however, it will be essential to verify the intracerebral stability (inhibited growth) of different primary cell types and achieve methods for monitoring the synthesis of the gene product in vivo.

As gene transfer techniques continue to develop, it is likely that genetic manipulation of neurons both in vitro and in vivo will become a more prominent focus of research. Genetically modified neurons would have distinct advantages over modified peripheral cells: in particular, they would most effectively integrate, both structurally and functionally, into a host brain. Such integration could be useful for

exploring the development of the CNS and the interactions between neural tissues.

For example, Renfranz et al. recently described the use of genetically modified neurons to explore the signals that may regulate cell-type differentiation in the brain [52]. Neurons obtained from the hippocampus of the fetal rat brain were infected with a retrovirus containing a temperature-sensitive oncogene. Cells that incorporated the transgene showed continued cellular proliferation at 33 °C but showed arrested growth and differentiation at 37 °C (body temperature). These modified neurons were then labeled with radioactive thymidine and implanted into the hippocampus or cerebellum of neonatal rats, two regions of the brain that show postnatal neurogenesis of granule cells. In both implantation sites, the immortalized hippocampal neurons appeared to cease dividing and were found mainly in association with granule cells of the dentate gyrus (hippocampus) or granule layer (cerebellum). Within these locations, the modified cells acquired neuronal morphologies, including axons and dendritic processes, which made them virtually indistinguishable from surrounding intrinsic granule cells. In addition, some of the immortalized cells implanted within the cerebellum appeared to develop into Bergmann glia, a cell type that is specific for the cerebellum. These results suggested that the grafted cells responded to endogenous, site-specific cues in the parenchymal environment that influenced cellular differentiation and positioning in the brain. More generally, this study reveals the usefulness of genetically modified cells as a tool for exploring basic issues concerning the development and plasticity of the CNS.

Ultimately, neurons in vivo will increasingly become targets of genetic modification. Breakefield and DeLuca recently reviewed some progress with the use of the herpes simplex virus for delivering genes to postmitotic neurons in vivo [8]. While this particular technique is still in a state of development, it is clear that methods for achieving somatic gene therapy will continue to be an area of intense investigation. Such techniques may eventually prove useful for treating CNS disease of genetic origin. However, the development of efficient in vivo gene transfer methods will resolve only one of a number of problems that arise in the quest for effective gene therapy in human genetic disorders: the dysfunctional gene must first be isolated and characterized, and the appropriate time and place for genetic intervention determined. Despite current limitations in gene transfer techniques, the integration of the methodology and experience of molecular biology into neuroscience research has provided, and will continue to provide, an intriguing new avenue for exploring the CNS and for conceptualizing, and developing, novel therapeutic approaches for the treatment of CNS diseases.

Acknowledgements. This research was supported by NIH AG06088, NIH AG08514, NIH AG10435, and the Margaret and Herbert Hoover Foundation. We thank M. L. Gage for assistance with the preparation of the manuscript.

References

1. Amaral DG, Kurz J (1985) An analysis of the origins of the cholinergic and noncholinergic septal projections to the hippocampal formation of the rat. J Comp Neurol 420: 37–59

2. Anderson KJ, Dam D, Lee S, Cotman CW (1988) Basic fibroblast growth factor prevents death of lesioned cholinergic neurons in vivo. Nature 332: 306–361

3. Appel SH (1981) A unifying hypothesis for the cause of amyotrophic lateral sclerosis, parkinsonism, and Alzheimer disease. Ann. Neurol 10: 499–505

4. Armstrong DM, Saper CB, Levey AI, Wainer BH, Terry BD (1983) Distribution of cholinergic neurons in rat brain demonstrated by the immunocytochemical localization of choline acetyltransferase. J Comp Neurol 216: 53–68

5. Barde YA, Edgar D, Thoenen H (1983) New neurotrophic factors. Annu Rev Physiol 45: 601–612

6. Bartus R, Dean RL, Beer C, Lippa AS (1982) The cholinergic hypothesis of geriatric memory dysfunction. Science 217: 408–417

7. Bjorklund A, Stenevi U (1981) In vivo evidence of a hippocampal adrenergic neurotrophic factor specifically release on septal deafferentation. Brain Res 229: 403–428

8. Breakefield XO, DeLuca NA (1991) Herpes simplex virus for gene delivery to neurons. New Biologist 3: 203–218

9. Brundin P, Isacson O, Bjorklund A (1985) Monitoring of cell viability in suspensions of embryonic CNS tissue and its use as a criterion for intracerebral graft survival. Brain Res 331: 251–259

10. Butcher LL (1983) Acetylcholinesterase histochemistry. In: Bjorklund A, Hokfelt T (eds) Handbook of chemical neuroanatomy, vol 1. Elsevier, Amsterdam, pp 1–49

11. Campenot RB (1982) Development of sympathetic neurons in compartmentalized cultures: I. Local control of neurite growth by nerve growth factors. Dev Biol 93: 1–12

12. Chen KC, Gage FH (1991) Nerve growth factor producing primary fibroblasts grafted into the basal forebrain of behaviorally characterized aged rats. Soc Neurosci Abstr 17: 1313

13. Collins F, Crutcher KA (1985) Neurothrophic activity in the adult rat hippocampal formation: regional distribution and increase after septal lesion. J Neurosci 5: 2809–2814

14. Collins F, Dawson A (1983) An effect of nerve growth factor on parasympathetic neurite outgrowth. Proc Natl Acad Sci USA 80: 2091–2094

15. Cowan WM, Fawcett JW, O'Leary DD, Stanfield BB (1984) Regressive events in neurogenesis. Science 225: 1258–1265

16. Coyle JT, Price DH, Delong MR (1983) Alzheimer's disease: a disorder of cortical cholinergic innervation. Science 219: 1184–1189

17. Culliton BJ (1989) ADA deficiency: a prime candidate. Science 246: 751

18. Edwards RH, Selby MJ, Rutter WJ (1986) Differential RNA splicing predicts two distinct nerve growth factor precursors. Nature 319: 784–787

19. Ernfors P, Ebendal T, Olson L, Mouton P, Strömberg I, Persson A (1989) A cell line producing recombinant nerve growth factor evokes growth responses in intrinsic and grafted central cholinergic neurons. Proc Natl Acad Sci USA 86: 4756–4760

20. Fisher LJ, Jinnah HA, Kale LC, Higgins GA, Gage FH (1991) Survival and function of intrastriatally grafted primary fibroblasts genetically modified to produce L-dopa. Neuron 6: 371–380

21. Fonnum F (1975) A rapid radiochemical method for the determination of choline acetyltransferase. J Neurochem 24: 407–409

22. Friedmann T (1989) Progress toward human gene therapy. Science 244: 1275–1281

23. Gage FH, Fisher LJ (1991) Intracerebral grafting: a tool for the neurobiologist. Neuron 6: 1–12

24. Gage FH, Bjorklund A, Stenevi U, Dunnett SB (1983) Functional correlates of compensatory collateral sprouting by aminergic and cholinergic afferents in the hippocampal formation. Brain Res 268: 39–47

25. Gage F, Wolff JA, Rosenberg MB, Xu L, Yee JE, Shults C, Friedmann T (1987) Grafting genetically modified cells to the brain: possibilities for the future. Neuroscience 23: 795–807

26. Gage FH, Bjorklund A (1986) Enhanced graft survival in the hippocampus following selective denervation. Neuroscience 17: 89–98

27. Gage FH, Wictorin K, Fischer W, Williams LR, Varon S, Bjorklund A (1986) Life and death of cholinergic neurons in the septal and diagonal band region following complete fimbria-fornix transection. Neuroscience 19: 241–255

28. Gospodarowicz D, Neufeld G, Schweigerer L (1986) Fibroblast growth factor. Mol Cell Endocrinol 46: 187–204

29. Grafstein B (1977) The nerve cell body response to axotomy. Exp Neurol 48: 32–51

30. Greene LA (1977) A quantitative bioassay for nerve growth factor (NGF) activity employing a clonal pheochromocytoma cell line. Brain Res 133: 350–353

31. Greene L, Shooter EM (1980) The nerve growth factor: biochemistry, synthesis, and mechanisms of action. Annu Rev Neurosci 3: 353–402

32. Gunderson RW, Barrett JN (1980) Characterizations of the turning response of dorsal root neurites toward nerve growth factor. J Cell Biol 87: 546–554

33. Hamburger V, Oppenheim RW (1982) Naturally occurring neuronal death in vertebrates. Neurosci Comment 1: 55–68

34. Hefti F (1986) Nerve growth factor (NGF) promotes survival of septal cholinergic neurons after fimbrial transections. J Neurosci 6: 2155–2162

35. Hefti F, Hartikka JJ, Eckenstein F, Gnahn H, Heumann R, Schwab M (1985) Nerve growth factor increases choline acetyl-transferase but not survival or fiber outgrowth of cultured fetal septal cholinergic neurons. Neuroscience 14: 55–68

36. Honegger P, Lenoir D (1982) Nerve growth factor (NGF) stimulation of cholinergic telencephalic neurons in aggregating cell cultures. Dev Brain Res 3: 229–238

37. Horellou P, Marlier L, Privat A, Mallet J (1990) Behavioral effect of engineered cells that synthesize L-dopa or dopamine after grafting into the rat neostriatum. Eur J Neurosci 2: 116–119

38. Horellou P, Brundin P, Kalen P, Mallet J, Bjorklund A (1990) In vivo release of DOPA and dopamine from genetically engineered cells grafted to the denervated rat striatum. Neuron 5: 393–402

39. Horellou P, Lundberg C, Brundin P, Wictorin K, Kalen P, Bjorklund A, Mallet J (1991) Genetic modification of primary glial cells with a human tyrosine hydroxylase gene 1. In vitro characterizations. Abstract from Foundation IPSEN meetings in Paris, 23.9.–24.9.1991

40. Katzman RN (1986) Alzheimer's disease. N Engl J Med 314: 964–973

41. Kawaja MD, Fagan AM, Firestein BL, Gage FH (1991) Intracerebral grafting of cultured autologous skin fibroblasts into the rat striatum: an assessment of graft size and ultrastructure. J Comp Neurol 307: 695–706

42. Kawaja MD, Fisher LJ, Schinstine M, Hyder J, Ray J, Chen LS, Gage FH (1992) Grafting genetically modified cells within the rat central nervous system: methodological considerations. In: Dunnett S, Bjorklund A (eds) Neural transplantation: a practical approach. Oxford University Press, Oxford, pp 21–55

43. Kawaja MD, Gage FH (1991) Primary fibroblasts genetically modified to produce nerve growth factor embedded within a collagen matrix act as a permissive graft for axonal regeneration in vivo. Soc Neurosci Abstr 17: 571

44. Leibrock J, Lottspeich F, Hohn A, Hofer M, Hengerer B, Masiakowski P, Thoenen H, Barde Y-A (1989) Molecular cloning and expression of brain-derived neurotrophic factor. Nature 341: 149–152

45. Lundberg G, Horellou P, Brundin P, Wictorin K, Kalen P, Mallet J, Bjorklund A (1991) Genetic modification of primary glial cells with a human tyrosine hydroxylase gene 2. In vivo grafting and function. Abstract from Foundation IPSEN meetings in Paris, 23.9.–24.9. 1991

46. Martinez HJ, Dreyfus CF, Jonakait GM, Black IB (1985) Nerve growth factor promotes cholinergic development in brain striatal cultures. Proc Natl Acad Sci USA 82: 7777–7781

47. McLoon LK, McLoon SC, Lund R (1981) Cultured embryonic retinae transplanted to rat brain: differentiation and formation of projections to host superior colliculus. Brain Res 226: 15–31
48. Mobley WC, Rutkowski JL, Tennekoon GI, Buchanan K, Johnston MW (1985) Choline acetyltransferase activity in striatum of neonatal rats increased by nerve growth factor. Science 229: 284–287
49. Morrison RS, Sharma A, DeVellis J, Bradshaw RA (1986) Basic fibroblast growth factor supports the survival of cortical neurons in primary culture. Proc Natl Acad Sci USA 83: 7537–7541
50. Nieto-Sampedro M, Manthorpe M, Barbin G, Varon S, Cotman CW (1983) Injury-induced neurotrophic activity in adult rat brain: correlation with survival delayed implants in wound cavity. J Neurosci 3: 2219–2229
51. Pearson RCA, Gatter KC, Powell TPS (1983) Retrograde cell degeneration in the basal nucleus of monkey and man. Brain Res 261: 321–326
52. Renfranz PJ, Cunningham MG, McKay RDG (1991) Region-specific differentiation of the hippocampal stem cell line HiB5 upon implantation into the developing mammalian brain. Cell 66: 713–729
53. Ronnett GV, Hester LD, Nye JS, Connors K, Snyder SH (1990) Human cortical neuronal cell line: establishment from a patient with unilateral megalencephaly. Science 248: 603–605
54. Rosenberg MB, Friedmann T, Robertson RC, Tuszynski M, Wolff JA, Breakefield XO, Gage FH (1988) Grafting genetically modified cells to the damaged brain: restorative effects of NGF expression. Science 242: 1575–1578
55. Satoh K, Armstrong DM, Fibiger HC (1983) A comparison of the distribution of central cholinergic neurons as demonstrated by acetylcholinesterase pharmacohistochemistry and choline acetyltransferase immunohistochemistry. Brain Res Bull 11: 693–720
56. Schinstine ML, Tosenberg MB, Routledge-Ward C, Whiting RL, Firedmann T, Gage FH (1992) Regulation of recombinant gene expression and ACh production by fibroblasts genetically modified to produce Drosophila choline acetyltransferase. J Neurochem 58: 2019–2029
57. Schwab ME, Otten U, Agid Y, Thoenen H (1979) Nerve growth factor (NGF) in the rat CNS: absence of specific retrograde axonal transport and tyrosine hydroxylase induction in locus ceruleus and substantia nigra. Brain Res 168: 473–483
58. Seiler M, Schwab ME (1984) Specific retrograde transport of nerve growth factor (NGF) from cortex to nucleus basalis in the rat. Brain Res 300: 33–39
59. Storm-Mathisen J (1974) Choline acetyltransferase and acetylcholinesterase in fascia dentata following lesions of the entorhinal afferent. Brain Res 80: 119–181
60. Thoenen H, Barde YA (1980) Physiology of nerve growth factor. Physiol Rev 60: 1284–1335
61. Thompson WG (1890) Successful brain grafting. N Y Med J 51: 701–702
62. Uchida K, Takamatsu K, Kaneda N, Toya S, Tsukada Y, Kurosawa Y, Fujita K, Nagatsu T, Kohsaka S (1989) Synthesis of L-3,4-dihydroxyphenylalamine by tyrosine hydroxylase cDNA-transfected C6 cells: application for intracerebral grafting. J Neurochem 53: 728–732
63. Ungerstedt U (1971) Striatal dopamine release after amphetamine or nerve degeneration revealed by rotational behavior. Acta Physiol Scand Suppl 367: 49–68
64. Walicke RS, Cowan WM, Ueno N, Baird A, Guillemin R (1986) Fibroblast growth factor promotes survival of dissociated hippocampal neurons and enhances neurite extension. Proc Natl Acad Sci USA 83: 3012–3015
65. Whitehouse PJ, Price DL, Struble RG, Clark AW, Coyle JT, DeLong MR (1982) Alzheimer's disease and senile dementia: loss of neurons in the basal forebrain. Science 215: 1237–1239
66. Williams LR, Varon S, Peterson GM, Wictorin K, Fischer W, Bjorklund A, Gage FH (1986) Continuous infusion of nerve growth factor prevents basal forebrain neuronal death after fimbriafornix transection. Proc Natl Acad Sci USA 83: 9231–9235
67. Wolff JA, Fisher LJ, Xu L, Jinnah HA, Langlais PJ, Iuvone PM, O'Malley KL, Rosenberg MB, Shimohama S, Friedmann T, Gage FH (1989) Grafting fibroblasts genetically modified to produce L-dopa in a rat model of Parkinson disease. Proc Natl Acad Sci USA 86: 9011–9014

Immunologic Aspects of Intracerebral CNS Tissue Transplantation

H. Widner

Restorative Neurology Unit, Department of Neurology, University Hospital, Lund, Sweden

Introduction

The development of intracerebral grafting (ICG) techniques intended to alleviate neurologic disorders has led to an increased interest in immune responses in the brain. In spite of the great advances made in the general understanding of such responses after transplantation of foreign tissues, a number of factors particularly important for immune responses within the central nervous system (CNS) still require elucidation. This chapter will review some of the mechanisms involved and describe some key findings on the immunologic constraints that are relevant for successful ICG.

General Aspects of Transplantation Immunology

The immune system has the ability to distinguish between self and non-self structures, the latter being called antigens. Antigen recognition is accomplished by B and T lymphocytes and their recognition molecules, the immunoglobulins and the T-cell receptors (TcRs). Immune responses against transplanted cells are elicited by genetically determined surface structures of the cells, called histocompatibility antigens. These molecules are polymorphic, i.e., there are numerous variants of them. The highest degree of difference between the individuals of a species is found within the major histocompatibility complex (MHC), the most important type of transplantation antigen. An individual's particular set of MHC molecules is unique, unless he or she has an identical twin. Transplantations of incompatible tissues or organs, i.e., with incompatible transplantation antigens, are called allogeneic (allografts) when made between different members of the same species and xenogeneic (xenografts) when made between different species. Immunologically incompatible tissues and organs that are transplanted to an immunologically competent host, i.e., an individual with an intact immune system, are at risk of being rejected. The survival of an allograft varies according to the degree of immunologic incompatibility, the size of the graft, and the implantation site.

It has been found that incompatible grafts survive longer at certain sites of the body, called immunologically privileged sites, than at others. The brain has been recognized as an immunologically privileged site. There are various definitions of the concept of immunologically privileged sites [2, 4, 18]. At such sites, at least one of the requirements for an immune response to occur against an allograft is not fulfilled [4].

The immune responses to a graft are probably best exemplified by homotopic skin grafts (Fig. 1). Tissues vary in their immunogenicity or ability to induce an immune response, partly because they contain differing numbers of antigen-presenting cells (APCs), i.e., cells that process and present the antigens. The skin has many specific APCs, called Langerhans cells, that normally circulate from the interstitial spaces of the skin via lymphatic vessels to regional lymph nodes. APCs carry antigens that have penetrated the skin to immunologically competent cells. This flow of cells constitutes the afferent arm of the immune response. If the APCs have taken up foreign antigens, partly degraded them (antigen processing), and incorporated the degraded products into their MHC molecules, there may be activation of T cells in lymph nodes. Activated T-helper cells (Th) expand in number and produce factors that make clonal expansion of B cells and T-killer cells (Tc) possible. The activated cells then migrate out of the lymph nodes and home to the graft, guided by adhesion molecules on the vessel walls; as a result, the cells in the graft will be killed. The migration and actions of effector cells constitute the efferent arm of the immune response.

The key difference between a specific immune response and a nonspecific inflammatory response is that in the former the lymphocytes are activated. This activation is very strictly regulated, so as not to give rise to untoward immune, e.g., autoimmune, responses. The activation of a T-helper cell results from the interaction between the lymphocyte and an APC (Fig. 2). There are specialized APCs (professional APCs) in most tissues, but they may vary in numbers and in their ability to present antigens. The APCs trap, partly degrade, and process antigens, and the resulting fragments are complexed with MHC class I or II molecules and expressed on the surface of the APC. When a TcR binds to

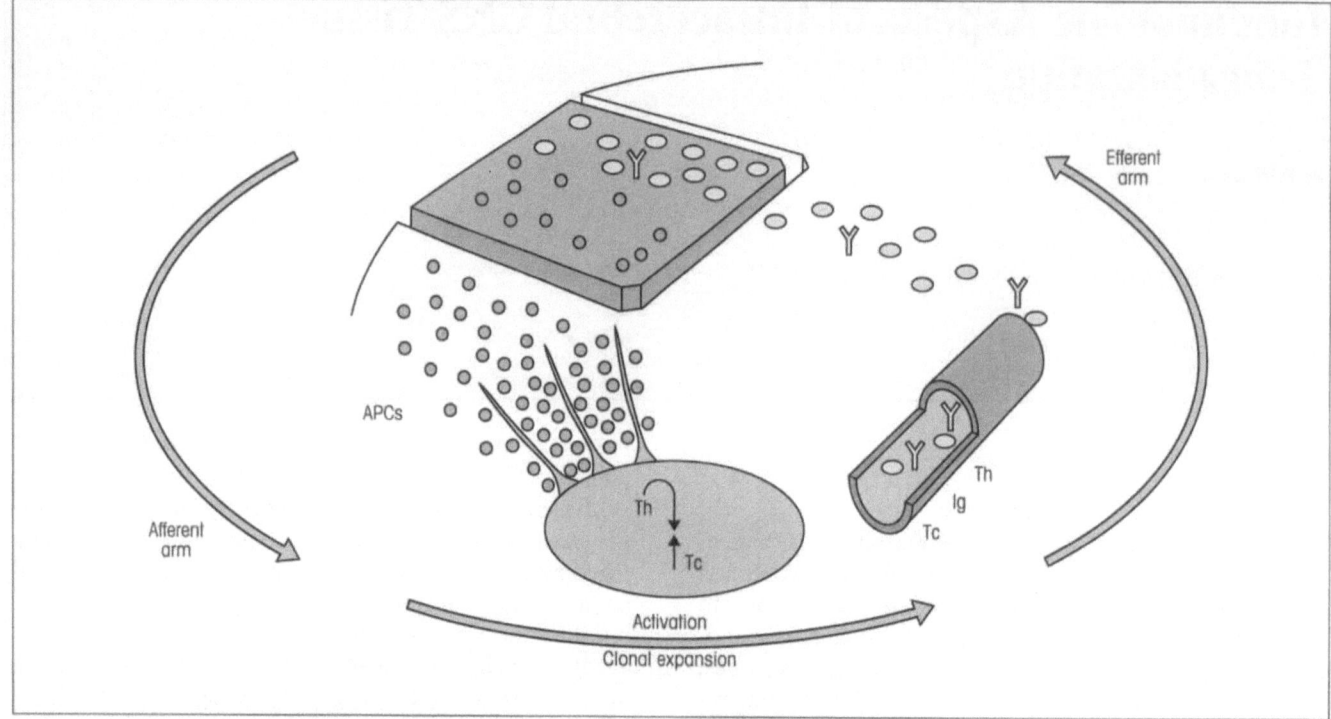

Fig. 1. Schematic outline of immunologic responses against a homotopic skin graft, i. e., a graft transplanted to the same location, skin to skin. The afferent arm comprises steps leading to immunization, i. e., activation of host lymphocytes and of effector mechanisms. Donor-derived specialized antigen-presenting cells (**APC**), called Langerhans cells in the skin, migrate from the skin graft to the regional lymph node draining the particular skin region. In the lymph node, T-helper cells (**Th**) are acti-vated and in turn help T-killer cells (**Tc**) to proliferate by supplying inter-leukin-2. T-helper cells also promote the activation of B cells, which start producing immunoglobulins, Ig (**Y**). In the efferent arm of the immune response, the activated antigen-specific cells and immunoglobulins pass into the blood circulation and home to the graft, via the mediation of cell-adhesion molecules

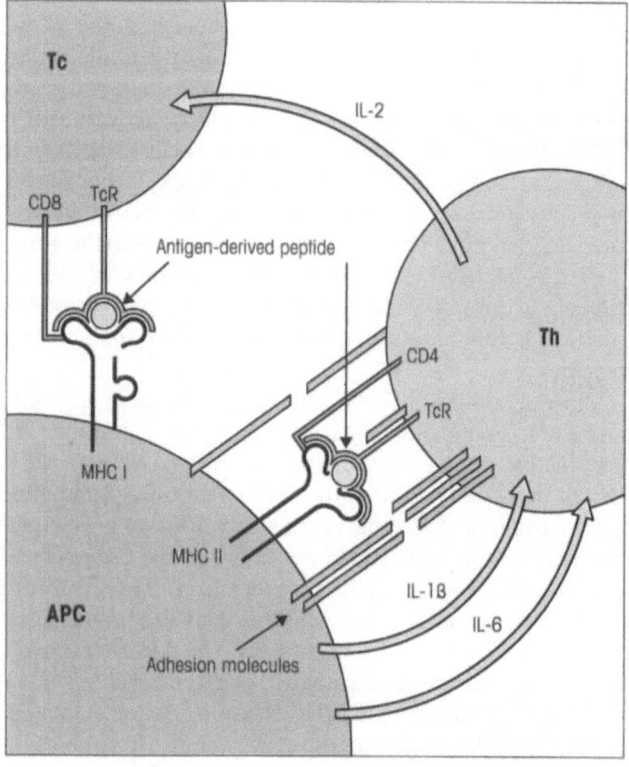

Fig. 2. Schematic illustration of the interactions between an antigen-pre-senting cell (**APC**), a T-helper cell (**Th**), and a T-killer cell (**Tc**). The APC takes up a protein antigen and degrades it into short peptide fragments that are integrated into major histocompatibility complex molecules of class I and II (**MHC I, MHC II**). T-helper cells bind to the MHC class II molecules via the accessory molecule CD4, whereas the T-cell receptor (**TcR**) binds to the MHC + peptide antigen complex on another part of the MHC molecule. The T-killer cells bind to the APC and target cell (in this instance one and the same cell) through interaction between the ac-cessory molecule CD8 and MHC class molecules and through TcR bind-ing to the MHC + peptide antigen complex. The binding between TcR and the MHC + peptide leads to initial activation signals, which are fol-lowed by additional activation signals mediated by other adhesion molecules between the APC and the Th (**hatched lines** between the **APC** and the **Th**). The APC also produces interleukin-1β (**IL-1β**) and/or in-terleukin-6 (**IL-6**), which support the early proliferation of the Th. The activated Th produces interleukin-2 (**IL-2**), which is a growth factor ab-solutely required for Th and Tc expansion

the MHC + antigen complex presented by the APC, there is a first signal transmitted to the lymphocyte, possibly through the CD3 stucture (cluster of differentiation-3 molecules) associated with the TcR, and possibly also through some other accessory molecules that may be able to transduce activation signals [21] (Fig. 3). The APCs also produce soluble factors, interleukin-1β (IL-1β) and interleukin-6 (IL-6), that increase the proliferation of the T-helper cells. The activation and further proliferation of T cells cannot occur in the absence of a growth factor produced exclusively by activated T-helper cells, interleukin-2 (IL-2), and unless there is at the same time a binding between the TcR and the MHC + antigen complex.

Activated lymphocytes leave the draining regional lymphatic tissue, enter the blood circulation, and are guided to the effector site by cues on the vascular epithelium, called addressins or adhesion molecules. Circulating lymphocytes have on their surface complementary binding structures called homing receptors. There are several such homing receptor-adressin pairs. These molecules guide the cells and regulate their interactions. The expression of addressins is induced on endothelial cells by cytokines such as γ-inter-

feron (γ-IFN), tumor necrosis factor α (TNF-α), IL-1, and IL-6 that are released in inflammatory responses [11, 12].

It has long been recognized that graft rejection in a host that receives a first transplant (previously unprimed recipient) is primarily a T-cell-mediated response [29]. However, virtually all components of the immune system may also be recruited later and participate in the destruction of the graft (Fig. 4). T-helper cells, cytotoxic T cells, macrophages, natural killer cells (NK cells), and antibodies are therefore often found within a rejected graft, but the initial and critical event for graft destruction is the activation of T-helper cells and cytotoxic T cells. In a previously primed recipient, antibodies play an important role in the initiation of the immune response. If MHC class I antibodies can be detected prior to the implantation, acute graft rejection is likely to occur [34].

Xenografts are often destroyed by preformed antibodies that bind to the grafted cells and in turn bind cells. Macrophages can subsequently attach via Fc receptors (immunoglobulin-binding receptors) to these antibodies. This leads to macrophage activation with release of cytotoxic products in a process called antibody-dependent cellular cytotoxicity (ADCC). Alternatively, these preformed anti-

Fig. 3. *Schematic close-up view of the interaction between an APC and a T-helper cell. The antigen-specific binding occurs between the* **TcR** *and the* **MHC** *molecule on the APC that has an antigenic peptide bound in its groove. The* **CD4** *(cluster of differentiation-4) molecule guides the binding of Th cells to MHC class II molecules. It is thought that, when there is specific binding between a TcR and an MHC + antigenic peptide, a large complex is formed with several TcRs and* **CD3** *(cluster of differentiation-3) molecules and this triggers an activation signal with Ca2+ influx. Additional activation signals may be mediated by other pairs of accessory molecules, such as* **LFA-3** *(leukocyte function antigen-3) and* **CD2***, and* **B7** *and* **CD28***. Additional intercellular adhesion is contributed by* **ICAM-1** *(immune cell adhesion molecule-1) and* **LFA-1** *molecules*

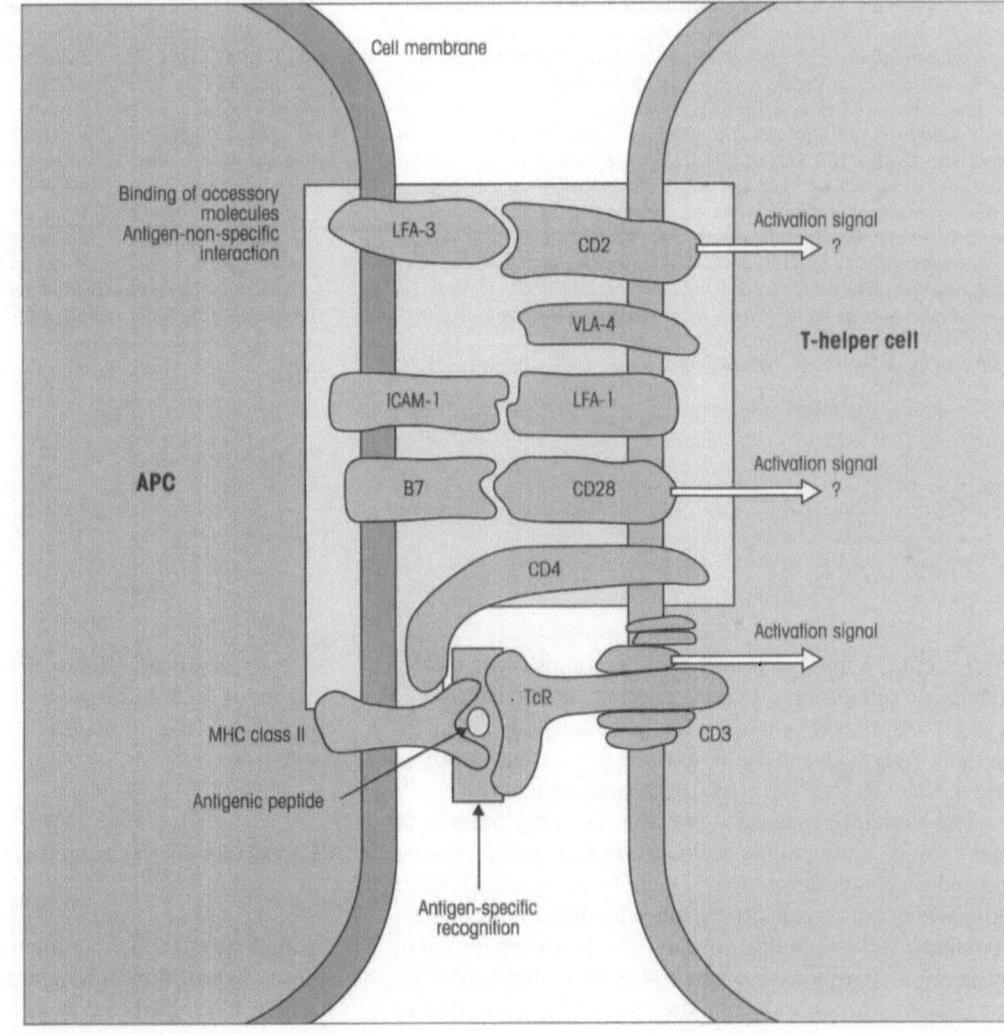

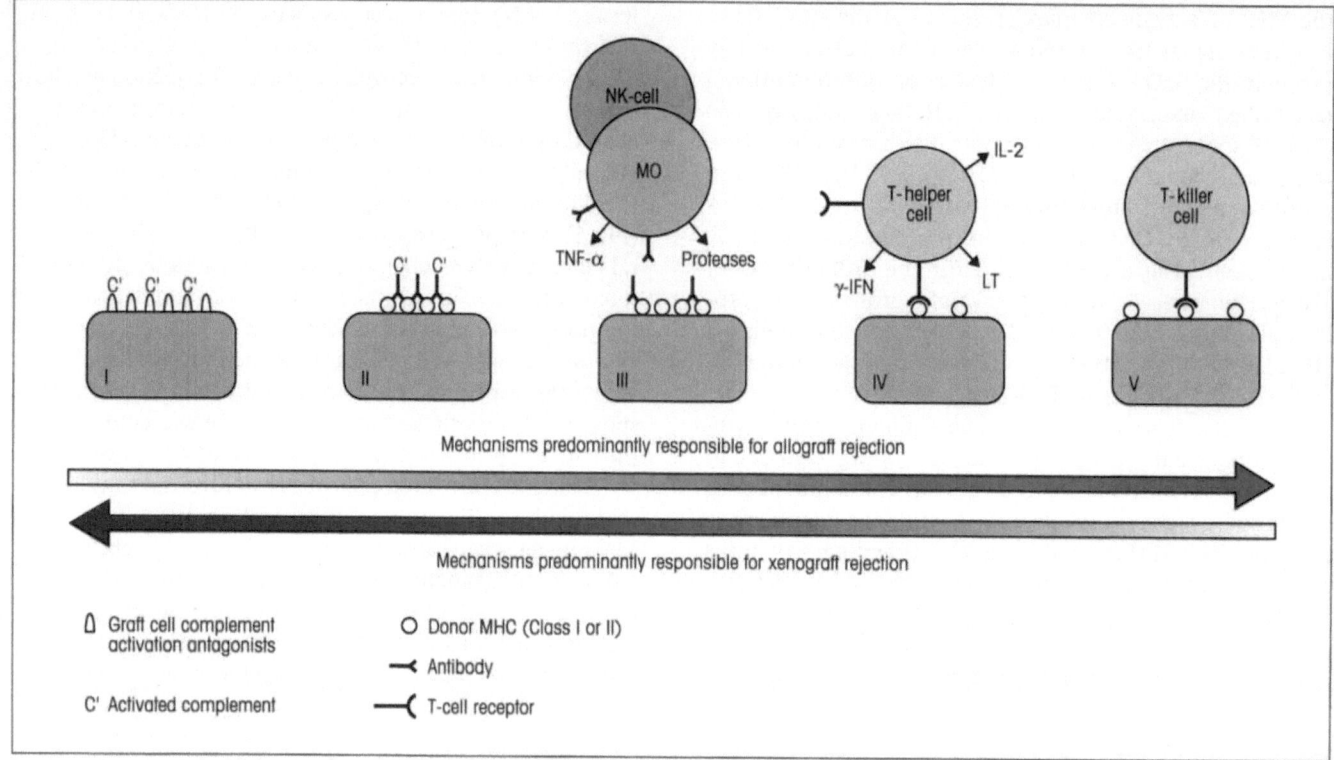

Fig. 4. *Schematic summary of possible mechanisms of immunologic graft rejection.* **I** *Direct complement activation occurs only in discordant xenograft situations, where the membrane-bound antagonists of complement activation on graft cells are incompatible with the host complement molecules that bind to the membrane of the graft cells.* **II** *Specific antibody binding to transplantation antigens and graft destruction by complement activation,* **C'**. *This type of response occurs in xenograft situations and in hyperacute rejection, e. g., in pre-immunized recipients in whom anti-HLA (antihuman leukocyte antigen) antibodies can be demonstrated prior to implantation.* **III** *Antibody-dependent cellular cytotoxicity, ADCC. Specific antibodies bind to the graft, and activated macrophages (**MO**) and other cells with Fc receptors bind to the antibodies and kill the graft via the release of mediators such as tumor necrosis factor α (**TNF-α**) and cytotoxic and tissue-damaging proteases. The role of the natural killer cell (**NK cell**) is unclear; it may act via ADCC.*
ADCC may occur in hyperacute rejection and responses to xenografts. **IV** *Specific interaction between graft cells and activated T-helper cells that produce cytotoxic substances such as γ-interferon (**γ-IFN**) and lymphotoxin (**LT** or TNF-β) and the growth factor interleukin-2 (**IL-2**), which is essential for other T lymphocytes. This type of response may occur against allografts and xenografts and may be part of a secondary inflammatory response, called delayed-type hypersensitivity, DTH. Collateral damage may occur as a consequence of the inflammation.* **V** *Specific interaction between a graft cell and an activated T-killer cell. The latter binds to the former and releases molecules, called perforins, that form pores in the target cell and cause its lysis. This specific interaction occurs in responses to allografts and also to some degree in responses to concordant xenografts. The **arrows** below the schematic drawings indicate what types of response are more likely to occur in responses to allografts and in responses to xenografts*

bodies bind to graft cells and activate complement factors that cause cellular lysis. Direct complement activation may occur in discordant xenografts as the consequence of an incompatibility between the donor-cell factors that suppress and the host factors that activate the complement cascade.

The immune response is specific, i.e., only those cells that express incompatible antigens are destroyed, whereas normal cells in their immediate vicinity are spared. T-killer cells lyse by cell-to-cell interaction, with little or no collateral damage to surrounding normal cells. However, if violent inflammatory responses occur, collateral damage may ensue, either through ischemia after vessel occlusion due to

the procoagulant effects of inflammation or through the effects of soluble cytotoxic factors released, for instance, by activated macrophages.

The Brain as a Transplantation Site

In analogy with the immune responses against a skin graft, those against immature neural tissue transplanted into the brain can be displayed as a circuit (Fig. 5). The present de-

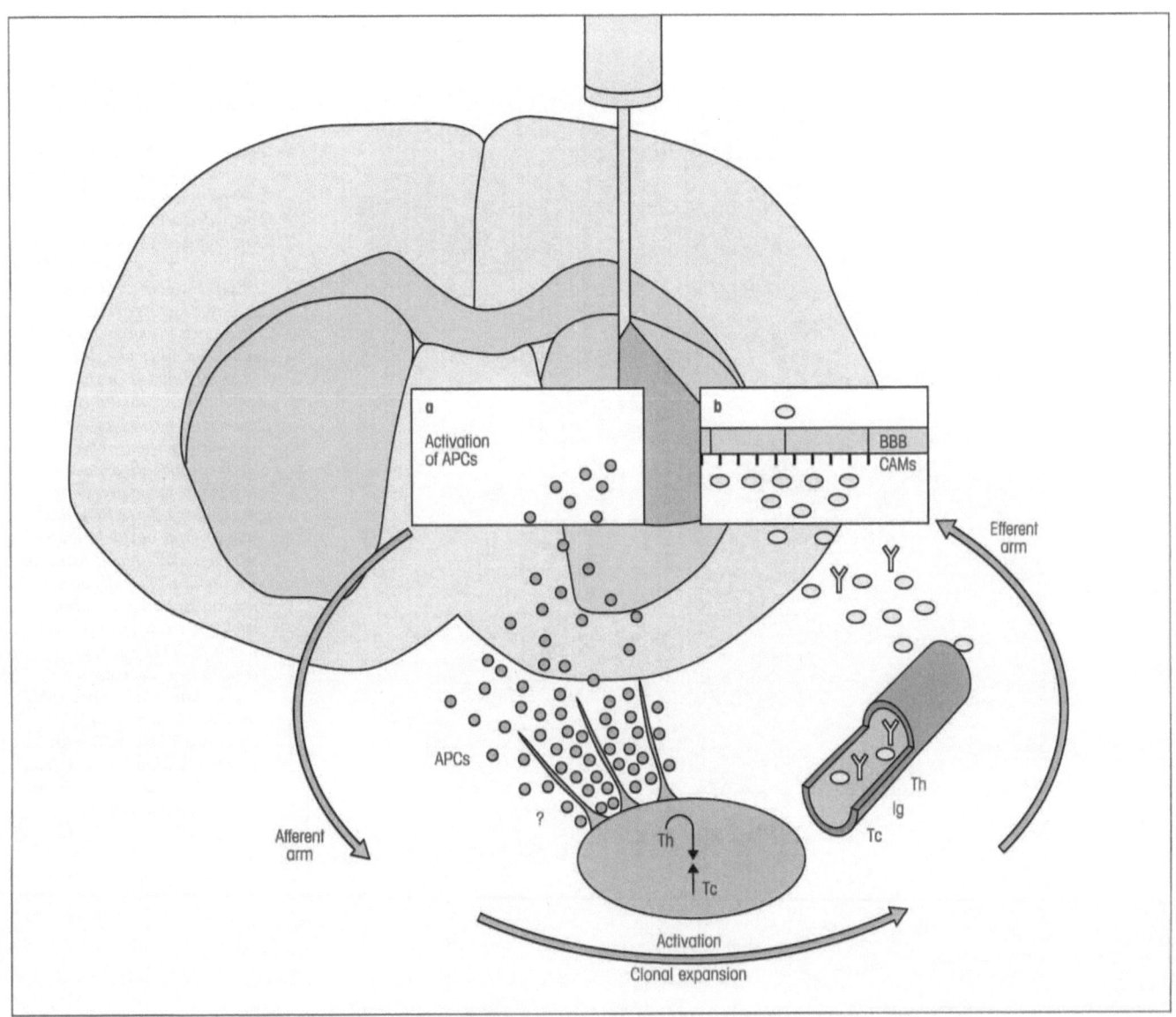

Fig. 5. Schematic outline of immunologic responses against a homotopic immature neural graft (graft transplanted to the same location: neural tissue to the brain). The afferent arm comprises steps leading to immunization, i. e., activation of host lymphocytes and effector mechanisms.
Donor-derived facultative antigen-presenting cells (**APCs**), probably astrocytes and microglia, may be activated and migrate from the brain graft
to regional lymphatic tissue, as summarized in **box a**. In a local/regional
lymphatic tissue, T-helper cells (**Th**) are activated and in turn help T-
killer cells (**Tc**) to proliferate. The anatomic location of the regional lymphatic tissue in relation to the human brain is unclear, as indicated by the
question mark. T-helper cells also promote the activation of B cells,
which start producing immunoglobulins, Ig (**Y**). In the efferent arm of
the immune response, the activated antigen-specific cells and immunoglobulins pass into the blood circulation and home to the graft, via
an interaction with cell-adhesion molecules (**CAM**) on the grafted endothelial cells. The passage of lymphocytes across the blood-brain barrier (**BBB**) is dependent on their state of activation (**box b**)

scription will focus on the cellular events that are thought to
occur when a semi-suspension of immature neuronal tissue
is implanted stereotaxically into the brain parenchyma; it is
based primarily on the experience gained in animal models
of Parkinson's disease (PD) and in patients with this disorder.

Donor Tissue Properties

For ICG into the rat model of PD, the donor tissue is the
ventral mesencephalic region [6]. The optimal donor age is
embryonic day E 13–15. The ventral mesencephalon from
one animal contains about 30000–40000 dopaminergic
(DA) neurons, i. e., 10 %–15 % of the total number of cells
(unpublished observations). The remaining cells and tissue
fragments are other types of neurons, glioblasts, intact vessels, free endothelial cells, microglia precursors, and remnants of the leptomeninges.

Brain-Derived Antigen-Presenting Cells

There are supposedly no dendritic cells (the most effective
APC type) or any other kind of professional APC in the

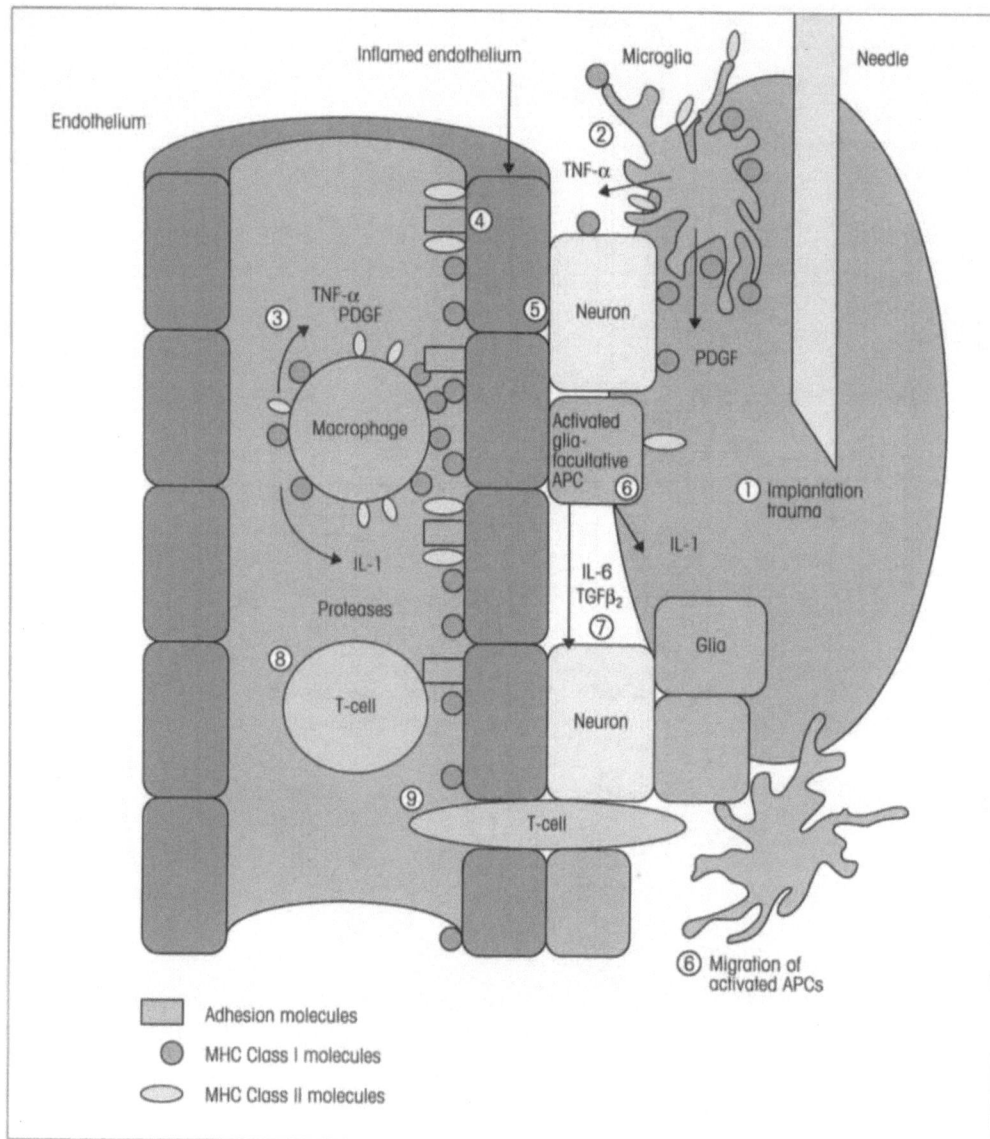

Fig. 6. Schematic drawing of the inflammatory events following a stereotaxic ICG of immature neural tissue. The brain tissue damage caused by the ICG (**1**) leads to the activation of host defense cells such as microglia (**2**) and blood-borne macrophages (**3**). These activated cells produce inflammatory mediators such as platelet-derived growth factor (**PDGF**), TNF-α, IL-1, and IL-6. These factors in turn induce an increased expression of cell-adhesion molecules on the endothelium (**4**) and graft cells and of transplantation antigens (MHC molecules) on graft cells (**5**). A proportion of the graft-derived glial cells are activated to become facultative antigen-presenting cells (**APCs**) that may migrate out of the graft area to regional lymphatic tissue (**6**). Production of locally acting immunosuppressive substances, such as transforming growth factor β₂ (TGFβ₂) may contribute to decrease the expression of MHC molecules on transplanted cells (**7**). Activated T cells adhere to the inflamed endothelium (**8**), pass the blood-brain barrier (**9**), and can kill the grafted cells

adult rodent brain [17]. However, there are other cells in the brain that express MHC class II antigens constitutively, e. g., cells along the ependyma and along the vessels in the white matter of adult rats [19]. Primordial microglial cells can be found in small clusters already from day E 16 in the fetal mouse brain. The microglia are the resident macrophages of the brain and constitute up to 13 % of the glial cells in the white matter [35]. They are phagocytic and can present antigens and activate T-helper cells after their own activation by γ-IFN [14]. There seem to be two lineages of microglial cells, namely those that enter the brain very early in ontogeny and those that enter the adult brain from the circulation. The latter are called perivascular microglial cells and are derived from the bone marrow [20].

Astrocytes are the most important component of connective tissue in the brain parenchyma. Resting astrocytes have virtually no immunologic activity, but astrocytes acti-

vated by γ-IFN and TNF-α can become APCs – i. e., they are facultative APCs – and express MHC class I and class II molecules, produce IL-1 and IL-6, and stimulate the proliferation of antigen-specific T-cell clones [45]. Astrocytes that are activated by the inflammatory response have a migratory capacity and can be found in the host brain at great distances from the implantation site [52]. If the cells enter the lymphatic system, they are likely to stimulate an immune response.

Donor-derived endothelial cells (ECs) too may function as APCs. γ-IFN induces increased levels of MHC class I antigens and de novo expression of class II antigens on ECs. It has not yet been demonstrated whether ECs from the cerebral circulation can produce IL-1 or IL-6, which is essential for them to act as effective APCs [39]. Such production has been demonstrated in ECs taken from vessels outside the brain [15].

In three recent ICG studies [23, 36, 37], host-derived microglial cells have been claimed to be the main APCs. This role proposed for host APCs in the initiation of allogeneic immune responses probably stems from the observation that host cells can present donor MHC molecules. However, host-derived APCs are far less able than donor-derived ones to evoke an immune response.

The number of donor- and possibly host-derived facultative APCs that are activated to functional APCs probably depends on the degree of local trauma caused by the ITP procedure.

Inflammatory Responses

The inflammatory response around a graft is triggered by a large number of potent substances released by systems that protect the body and participate in repair mechanisms. What systems are activated and the relative amount of inflammatory stimuli that is generated is at least partly proportional to the degree of tissue damage caused by graft implantation. IL-1β or IL-6 is released by most cells in response to damage; these cytokines are not only chemotactic for monocytes and macrophages, but they also activate these cells. The activated cells release a cascade of cytokines such as TNF-α, IL-1, IL-6, and platelet-derived growth factor (PDGF). Some of these cytokines can induce adhesion molecules and MHC molecule expression. The cytokines coordinate the various cellular responses involved in inflammation and immune responses [1] (Fig. 6).

Major Histocompatibility Complex Regulation in Grafted Tissue In Situ

Brain cells normally express very low levels of MHC antigens, if at all. Only certain cells, such as the endothelial cells, perivascular cells, microglia, and connective tissue cells, express MHC class I molecules. In addition, microglia and astrocytes have the potential to express MHC class II antigens. Why neurons and glia in the CNS normally have only weak expression of MHC molecules is unknown.

There is evidence of an increased expression of MHC antigens on grafted fetal CNS tissue. Even in a syngeneic, or isogeneic, situation – i.e., when the donor and the recipient have identical genotypes (the graft is then called a syngraft) – there is slightly increased expression of MHC on grafted and host cells [30], indicating that the implantation trauma causes MHC expression. More pronounced MHC expression has been shown in allografts and xenografts [46].

It is not known yet whether all cells in a graft can express MHC class I and class II antigens, and no studies performed to date have clearly demonstrated MHC class II antigen expression on neurons. Only γ-IFN and TNF-α have so far been shown to increase the expression of MHC on brain cells in vitro. The cellular source of γ-IFN is generally thought to be activated T cells. TNF-α can be released by activated macrophages, microglia, and astrocytes.

Regional Lymphatic Tissue

The explanation most commonly given for the fact that immune responses are impaired in the brain is the absence of lymphatic vessels in this organ [51]. However, the deduction that there is no direct passage of fluid or particles from the brain parenchyma to the lymphatics is erroneous. If radioactive macromolecular material is injected into the caudate nucleus of rabbits, 50% of the radioactivity can be recovered in the deep cervical lymph nodes [3]. In rodents, there are two major drainage routes of cerebrospinal fluid (CSF): through the arachnoidal villi and across the cribriform plate. After passage through the cribriform plate, antigens enter lymphatics in the neck. The intracerebral fluid drainage routes, which connect to the normal lymphatic system, can be called prelymphatics. Antigen injection into the forebrain produces a localized immune response in the deep cervical lymph nodes in rodents [16, 49]. The intracerebral injection of lymphochoriomeningitis virus into mice leads in the deep cervical lymph nodes to a proliferation of Tc cells that precedes a subsequent immunologic attack on the brain [10].

In cats and monkeys with increased intracranial pressure, a small proportion of CSF is transported to regional lymph nodes [28, 31]. However, drainage of CSF and brain interstitial fluid into regional lymphatic tissue has not been demonstrated in higher species with normal intracranial pressure. The possible role of cervical lymph nodes as amplification sites for immune responses in the human brain is consequently unknown.

In chronic inflammatory processes such as multiple sclerosis, the transformation of perivascular spaces into lymphatic tissue has been described. The cells in these perivascular spaces are then capable of mounting all types of immune response and may in fact function as regional lymphatic tissue [38]. The perivascular spaces are also a site for resident microglia, and bone-marrow-derived microglia and monocytes regularly enter and leave these spaces [20]. The filtering and processing of brain-derived antigens could take place in the perivascular spaces. Blood-derived APCs could leave these spaces to reach a lymphatic tissue somewhere outside the brain and mount a very effective immune response against the graft.

Graft Vascularization and Blood-Brain Barrier Formation

There are currently seven cloned substances capable of inducing angiogenesis. Of these, TNF-α, transforming growth factor α (TGF-α), acidic fibroblast growth factor (aFGF), and basic fibroblast growth factor (bFGF) can be produced locally in the brain in response to injury and inflammation. Several of these factors have mitogenic effects on glial cells.

Fetal neural tissue is vascularized from the periphery, and a vascular net is formed early in ontogeny. Solid pieces of immature donor tissue contain vessels already formed that can hook up to nearby host vessels, and it has been shown that vessels in solid grafts are almost exclusively of donor origin. During the preparation of cell suspensions of donor tissue, however, the vessels are disrupted. Thus, one can expect that the vessels in the graft are largely derived from the host, as angiogenesis seems to proceed from intact vessels. By means of monoclonal antibodies to various MHC antigens, it has been shown (unpublished observation) that in mouse allografts the vessels are made up by a mosaic of host- and donor-derived ECs.

The blood-brain barrier (BBB) consists of several components: (1) a physical barrier complex, which comprises a low pinocytic capacity in the cerebral EC, an electric potential difference between the luminal and aluminal surfaces, specialized transporters for certain substances, and a complex of dense intercellular connections (tight junctions); and (2) an enzymatic barrier complex of degrading enzymes within the EC.

The BBB properties are induced by astrocytes, as has been demonstrated in the iris, in which blood vessels acquire BBB functions after astrocytes have been injected into the anterior chamber of the eye [22]. The BBB complex is normally formed during embryonic and early perinatal life. It has been shown in animal experiments that intracerebral neural grafts establish a well-developed physical and enzymatic BBB within 1–2 weeks after ICG [5, 7, 41], and the vessels exhibit an enzymatic barrier [42]. Nonneuronal tissues (e. g., adrenal medulla) grafted to the CNS do not form a BBB.

Lymphocyte Passage Across the Blood-Brain Barrier

The normal brain parenchyma is virtually devoid of lymphocytes. However, lymphocytes can home to the CNS during various disease states [9]. Ligands for homing structures are present on cerebral ECs after induction, for example, by γ-IFN. Activated lymphocytes have been shown to pass the BBB irrespective of antigen specificity [45]. The relative effectiveness of this passage, i. e., the proportion of activated lymphocytes that enter the brain, is unknown but is lower than in other tissues. It is not known whether MHC expression plays a role in this passage [43, 44]. It has been suggested that NK cells are restricted from entering the brain parenchyma. NK cells have been proposed to eliminate cells devoid of MHC expression, and their presence in brain would thus be deleterious. Indeed, tumor cells devoid of MHC are cleared from the periphery [27] but not from the brain. In contrast, tumor cells with MHC expression are cleared from both the brain and the periphery.

Locally Produced Immunosuppressive Factors

Locally produced factors with immunosuppressive activity, i. e., that decrease MHC expression or minimize lymphocyte migration through the brain parenchyma, have been postulated. In the immature, but not in the adult, brain, α-fetoprotein is believed to decrease immune reactivity, mainly by reducing the expression of MHC class II molecules. How-

ever, even if fetal donor tissue can produce α-fetoprotein, it seems unlikely that the small number of cells implanted can produce enough of it to ensure a prolonged graft survival.

Prostaglandin E_2 (PGE_2) and transforming growth factor β_2 (TGF-β_2) are produced by activated astrocytes. TGF-β_2 ist claimed to be immunosuppressive, and it has been suggested that certain patients with gliomas have an impaired immune status owing to the high levels of TGF-β_2 produced by their tumors. The immunosuppressive mechanism of action of TGF-β_2 is unclear, but it possibly has antiproliferative effects.

Immunologic Experiences of Intracerebral Transplantation in Animals

The concept of the brain as an immunologically privileged site is often misinterpreted as implying indefinite graft survival. Immune responses can occur in the brain, even though components of the immune response can be less active than elsewhere in the body. Intracerebral transplants in rodents and nonhuman primates have shown a variable degree of survival, and no simple conclusion can be drawn from the results obtained [46]. Besides, the level of immunosuppression necessary in patients cannot be deduced from animal experiments, for there are pronounced quantitative differences between species in the capacity of the immune system. Certain general principles, however, can be established on the basis of animal experiments.

ICG to strongly pre-immunized hosts invariably leads to rejection of transplants [32], proof that the brain cannot shield a graft under all circumstances. Without immunosuppression, allografts can survive for a long time in the brain [30, 48], but they can also be rejected [23, 30, 33]. Most intracerebral transplants to nonhuman hosts have been performed without chronic immunosuppression, and long-term functional responses have been observed [e. g., 13]. Yet, little information on between-group differences is available, and it is unknown whether immunosuppression would have ensured the preservation of larger grafts and their having greater effects. Not only may preimmunization by a first intracerebral allograft cause a second intracerebral allograft to be rejected [47], but also the first intracerebral graft may be jeopardized by a second graft, as has been observed in primates [13]. These experiments demonstrate the existence of both an afferent and an efferent arm to the immune response in the brain. Xenografts have a poorer survival rate than allografts, but occasionally they seem to survive unimpaired [7, 30]. Technical aspects probably play a major role in the outcome of ICGs: for instance, tissue pieces seem to survive less well in the ventricles than in the brain parenchyma [40].

Prolonged Graft Survival in the Brain

Results from animal experiments enable a hypothetical scenario to be drawn for the cellular events that follow ICG of

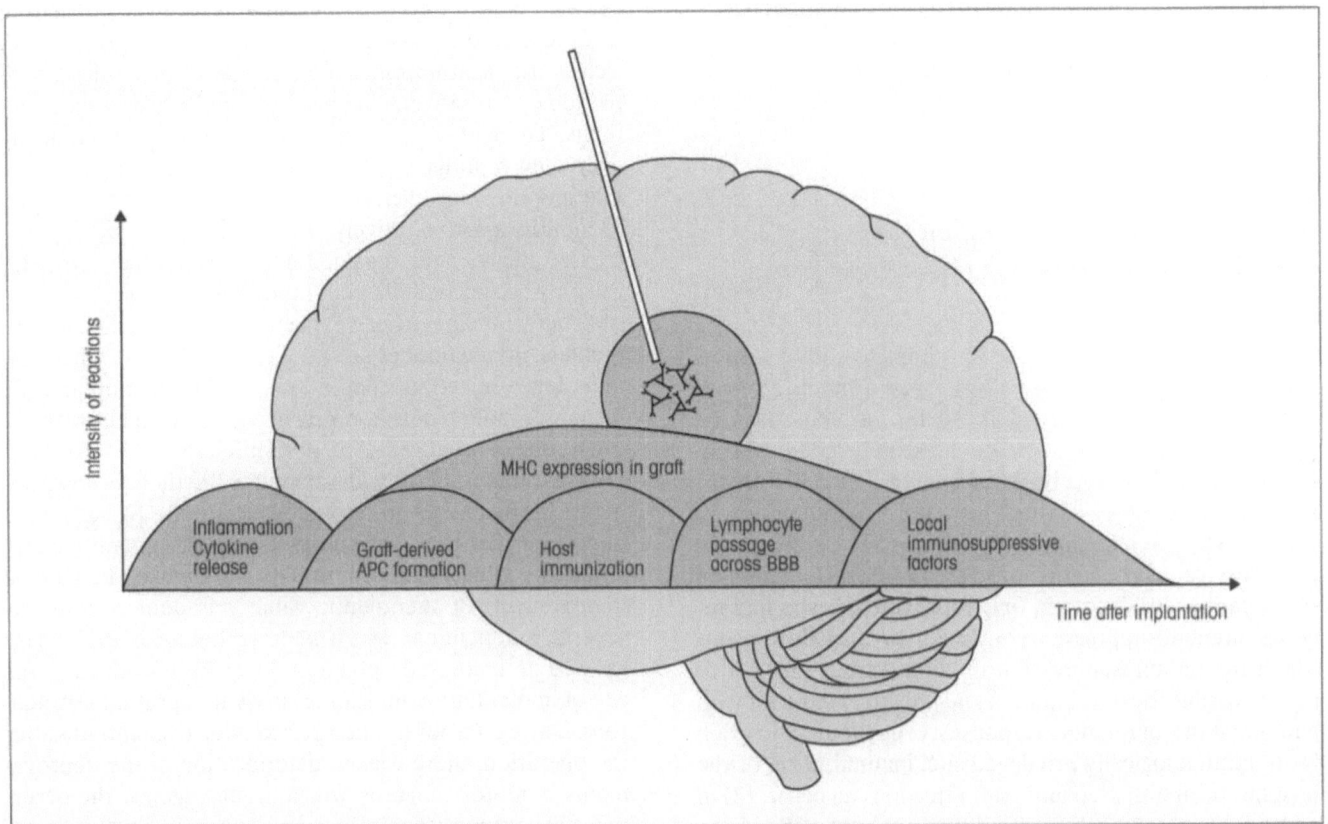

Fig. 7. *Proposed sequence of events after ICG of immature neural tissue and schematic representation of the intensity and duration of immunologic responses. The implantation trauma leads to the release of cytokines from nonspecific host defense cells, which in turn leads to the induction of graft-derived facultative antigen-presenting cells and the expression of donor-type MHC on the grafted cells. The APCs may induce a specific immunologic response, with host immunization (lympho-* *cyte proliferation) in regional lymphatic tissue or possibly in the brain parenchyma. The passage across the blood-brain barrier depends on the degree of induction of adhesion molecules on the vessels and the activation status of the lymphocytes. Finally, the duration of the expression of MHC molecules depends on the amount of stimulatory and inhibitory cytokines that are produced in the graft area*

fetal neural tissue (Fig. 7). There are three different kinds of donor- and host-derived APC, with differing immunization capabilities. The strongest immunizing stimulus is donor-derived, professional APCs expressing MHC class II antigens. The number of these cells depends on the amount of subpial and meningeal structures included in the donor tissue. ICG leads to local trauma and inflammation, and the number of facultative donor APCs activated depends on how intense and sustained the inflammatory response is. Induced donor MHC structures are shed and processed by host APCs. These three kinds of APC may migrate to regional lymphatic tissue, in proportion to the duration and intensity of the inflammatory stimulus. The activation of lymphocytes specific for an allogeneic antigen occurs in part in proportion to the number of APCs that reach the lymphatic tissue and the duration of their effect. The activated lymphocytes then enter the blood circulation.

The number of activated lymphocytes that home to the graft depends on several factors, the inflammatory response

at the graft site playing a major role: it induces angiogenesis and an increased number of adhesion molecules on the luminal side of the ECs, which, if graft-derived, may express allogeneic MHC molecules. The number of adhesion molecules and allogeneic MHC molecules is determined by the intensity and duration of the inflammatory response. The likelihood of activated lymphocytes' homing to the graft area is roughly proportional to the area of inflamed donor and host vasculature. The area of inflamed donor-derived vasculature is larger in a solid tissue graft than in a graft prepared as a suspension. Besides, the implantation trauma is smaller and the duration of inflammatory stimuli shorter with suspension grafts. Fewer activated allospecific lymphocytes are needed to provoke the rejection of a solid than of a suspension graft.

The final step in graft destruction is the recognition of the target cells by the cytotoxic T cells, which ultimately depends on the expression of donor MHC molecules on the surface of the grafted cells. This is influenced to a large extent by the degree and duration of the inflammation, but locally produced immunomodulatory factors that decrease MHC expression may play an important role.

Immunologic Experience of Intracerebral Transplantation in Patients with Parkinson's Disease

The ICG of fetal neural tissue into humans with disorders such as Parkinson's disease (PD) raises a number of immunologic questions. There is, so far, no consensus on whether immunosuppression should be used. About 100 patients with PD have received transplants of human fetal tissue, and some 30–40 of them have not been immunosuppressed. However, no simple conclusion can be drawn, since graft survival has been demonstrated by positron emission tomography (PET) scan in only four patients, who had received immunosuppression [25, 26, 50]. In short, the reasons for using immunosuppression in clinical trials are: (1) to make possible the development and growth of the graft with a minimal risk of immune responses; even though the brain is an immunologically privileged site, immunization of the host has been observed and graft rejection can occur; (2) in order not to preclude the possibility of a second graft, whose survival would be jeopardized in a pre-immunized recipient; finally, (3) to reduce the risk of adverse, though unlikely, autoimmune responses.

There are several ways of reducing the long-term risk for graft rejection. Pharmacologic treatment should be directed against inflammatory stimuli and factors that can generate host defense cells. Steroids are the most potent antiinflammatory compounds available; they decrease the amount of released IL-1, TNF-α, and other potent mediators, mainly by inhibiting macrophage activation. Drugs affecting other components of the inflammatory response, e.g., indomethacin and other prostaglandin inhibitors, cannot be used because of their anticoagulant effects. Since not all inflammatory stimuli are likely to be controlled by steroid treatment, temporary treatment with drugs that inhibit T-cell activation and proliferation are most likely to be beneficial. Ciclosporin (also known as cyclosporin A) is a potent inhibitor of T-cell activation, and azathioprine has antimitotic effects and can to some extent prevent a rapid proliferation of lymphocytes and macrophages. The toxicity of the compounds can be reduced considerably by combining them. A triple-drug regimen (ciclosporin, azathioprine, and steroids) has become widely used for kidney graft recipients [8].

Other ways of reducing the immune responses in a clinical situation, without the need for chronic immunosuppression, may consist in eliminating donor-derived APCs or specifically interfering with the initiation steps of the immune responses and with homing processes.

Our own first attempt to graft ventral mesencephalic tissue from human fetuses into the striata of two patients with PD was made in 1987 [24]. The patients received tissue from three to four fetuses each and were immunosuppressed with ciclosporin, azathioprine, and steroids. Only moderate improvement of movement speed was observed in these patients. The gait of the second patient improved gradually over a few months, and the improvement persisted for several months. However, during two short episodes, 11 and 13 months postoperatively, these benefits suddenly decreased and were not regained. The cause for these episodes can only be speculated upon. Immunologic rejection is possible but would have been expected to occur earlier. Unfortunately, no techniques are available for diagnosing an immunologic rejection. While suggesting an immunologic response, sudden deterioration in a graft recipient with PD can be due to other causes, e.g., an infection.

Two other patients with idiopathic PD then received implants by means of an improved technique [25, 26]. One important change was the use of a smaller implantation instrument, which reduced the local damage. Functional improvement of therapeutic value was demonstrated by several independent assessment techniques. PET scans showed an increased uptake of 6-L-[^{18}F]fluorodopa at the site of implantation, indicating survival of grafted DA neurons. During the observation period of up to 14 months after the operation, there was no deterioration of the improvements in motor function, which argues against the occurrence of immune rejection.

Two patients with parkinsonism induced by the toxic substance MPTP have received bilateral intrastriatal implants, with a 2-week interval between operations. There has been a progressive therapeutic improvement in both patients, with decreased muscular rigidity, increased movement speed, and less severe and fewer side effects of the antiparkinsonian medication. The improvements have been paralleled by an increased fluorodopa uptake in PET scans. Both patients were immunosuppressed with the triple-drug regimen; ciclosporin was gradually withdrawn after 12 months, and azathioprine after 18 months, but steroid treatment goes on. At 22 and 24 months after the operation, there has been no sign of graft rejection; on the contrary, the patients' clinical condition has continued to improve, even after the reduction in immunosuppressive treatment [50].

Conclusions

Immune responses do not seem to be a major hindrance for graft survival in animal and human brains, and short-term immunosuppressive treatment may be adequate to ensure graft survival. However, the ICG techniques used must be optimized so as to reduce to a minimum the events that can trigger immune responses. A better knowledge of the kinetics of immune responses against immature neural tissue and of the cellular mechanisms involved in them will make possible more specific interference with events leading to immune rejection.

Acknowledgements. The work was supported in part by grants from the Swedish Medical Research Council, the Faculty of Medicine, University of Lund, the Hardebo Foundation, and Schmitz's Foundation. The illustrations were designed by Håkan Widner and Bengt Mattson.

References

1. Arai K-I, Lee F, Mayajima A, Miyatake S, Arai N, Yokota T (1990) Cytokines: coordinators of immune and inflammatory responses. Annu Rev Biochem 59: 783–836

2. Barker CF, Billingham RE (1977) Immunologically privileged sites. Adv Immunol 25: 1–52

3. Bradbury MW, Westrop RJ (1983) Factors influencing exit of substances from cerebrospinal fluid into deep cervical lymph of the rabbit. J Physiol (Lond) 339: 519–534

4. Brent L (1990) Immunologically privileged sites. In: Johansson BB, Owman C, Widner H (eds) Pathophysiology of the blood-brain barrier. Long term consequences of barrier dysfunction for the brain. Elsevier, Amsterdam, pp 383–402 (Fernström Foundation series, 14)

5. Broadwell RD, Charlton HM, Balin BJ, Salcman M (1987) Angioarchitecture of the CNS, pituitary gland, and intracerebral grafts revealed with peroxidase cytochemistry. J Comp Neurol 260: 47–62

6. Brundin P, Björklund A, Lindvall O (1990) Practical aspects of the use of human fetal brain tissue for intracerebral grafting. Prog Brain Res 82: 707–714

7. Brundin P, Widner H, Nilsson OG, Strecker RE, Björklund A (1989) Intracerebral xenografts of dopamine neurons: the role of immunosuppression and the blood-brain barrier. Exp Brain Res 75: 195–207

8. Brynger H, Persson H, Flatmark A et al. (1988) No effect of blood transfusions or HLA matching on renal graft success rate in recipients treated with cyclosporin-prednisolone or cyclosporin-azathioprine-prednisolone: the Scandinavian experience. Transplant Proc 20 [suppl 3]: 261–263

9. Cross AH, Cannella B, Brosnan CF, Raine CS (1990) Homing to central nervous system vasculature by antigen-specific lymphocytes: I. Localization of ^{14}C-labeled cells during acute, chronic and relapsing experimental allergic encephalitis. Lab Invest 63: 162–170

10. Doherty PC, Allen JE, Lynch F, Ceredig R (1990) Dissection of an inflammatory process induced by CD8$^+$ T cells. Immunol Today 11: 55–59

11. Dujivestijn AM, Schreiber AB, Butcher EC (1986) Interferon-γ-regulates an antigen specific for endothelial cells involved in lymphocyte traffic. Proc Natl Acad Sci USA 83: 9114–9118

12. Dustin ML, Rothlein R, Bhan AK, Dinarello CA, Springer TA (1986) Induction by IL-1 and interferon-γ: tissue distribution and function of a natural adherence molecule (ICAM-1). J Immunol 137: 245–254

13. Freed CR, Richards JB, Sabol KE, Reite ML (1988) Fetal substantia nigra transplants lead to dopamine cell replacement and behavioral improvement in bonnet monkeys with MPTP induced parkinsonism. In: Beart PM, Woodruff GN, Jackson DM (eds) Pharmacology and function of dopaminergic neurons. Macmillan, London, pp 353–360

14. Frei K, Siepl C, Groscurth P, Bodmer S, Schwerdel C, Fontana A (1987) Antigen presentation and tumor cytotoxicity by interferon-γ-treated microglial cells. Eur J Immunol 17: 1271–1278

15. di Giovini FS, Duff GW (1990) Interleukin-1: the first interleukin. Immunol Today 11: 13–19

16. Harling-Berg C, Knopf PM, Merriam J, Cserr HF (1989) Role of cervical lymph nodes in the systemic humoral immune response to human serum albumin microinfusion into rat cerebrospinal fluid. J Neuroimmunol 25: 185–193

17. Hart DNJ, Fabre JW (1981) Demonstration and characterization of Ia-positive dendritic cells in the interstitial connective tissues of rat heart and other tissues, but not brain. J Exp Med 154: 347–361

18. Head JR, Billingham RE (1985) Immunologically privileged sites in transplantation immunology and oncology. Perspect Biol Med 29: 115–131

19. Head JR, Griffin WS (1985) Functional capacity of solid tissue transplants in the brain: evidence for immunological privilege. Proc R Soc Lond [Biol] 224: 375–387

20. Hickey WF, Kimura H (1988) Perivascular microglial cells of the CNS are bone-marrow derived and present antigen in vivo. Science 239: 290–292

21. Janeway CA (1989) The role of CD4 in T-cell activation: accessory molecule or co-receptor? Immunol Today 10: 234–238

22. Janzer RC, Raff MC (1987) Astrocytes induce blood-brain barrier properties in endothelial cells. Nature 325: 253–257

23. Lawrence JM, Morris RJ, Wilson DJ, Raisman G (1990) Mechanisms of allograft rejection in the rat brain. Neuroscience 37: 431–462

24. Lindvall O, Rehncrona S, Brundin P, Gustavii B, Astedt B, Widner H, Lindholm T, Björklund A, Leenders KL, Rothwell JC, Frackowiak R, Marsden CD, Johnels B, Steg G, Freedman R, Hoffer BJ, Seiger A, Bygdeman M, Strömberg I, Olson L (1989) Human fetal dopamine neurons grafted into the striatum in two patients with severe Parkinson's disease: a detailed account of methodology and a 6 months follow-up. Arch Neurol 46: 615–631

25. Lindvall O, Brundin P, Widner H, Rehncrona S, Gustavii B, Frackowiak R, Leenders KL, Sawle G, Rothwell JC, Marsden CD, Björklund A (1990) Grafts of fetal dopamine neurons survive and improve motor function in Parkinson's disease. Science 247: 547–574

26. Lindvall O, Widner H, Rehncrona S, Brundin P, Odin P, Gustavii B, Frackowiak R, Leenders KL, Sawle G, Rothwell JC, Björklund A, Marsden CD (1992) Transplantation of fetal dopamine neurons in Parkinson's disease: 1-year clinical and neurophysiological observations in two patients with putaminal implants. Ann Neurol 31: 155–165

27. Ljunggren H-G, Yamasaki T, Collins P, Klein G, Kärre K (1988) Selective acceptance of MHC class I-deficient tumor grafts in the brain. J Exp Med 167: 730–735

28. Love JA, Leslie RA (1984) The effects of raised ICP on lymph flow in the cervical lymphatic trunks in cats. J Neurosurg 60: 577–581

29. Mason DW, Morris PJ (1986) Effector mechanisms in allograft rejection. Annu Rev Immunol 4: 119–145

30. Mason DW, Charlton HM, Jones AJ, Lavy CB, Puklavec M, Simmonds SJ (1986) The fate of allogeneic and xenogeneic neuronal tissue transplanted into the third ventricle of rodents. Neuroscience 19: 685–694

31. McComb JG, Hyman S (1990) Lymphatic drainage of cerebrospinal fluid in the primate. In: Johansson BB, Owman C, Widner H (eds) Pathophysiology of the blood-brain barrier. Long term consequences of barrier dysfunction for the brain. Elsevier, Amsterdam, pp 421–438 (Fernström Foundation series 14)

32. Medawar PB (1948) Immunity to homologous grafted skin: III. The fate of skin homografts transplanted to the brain, to subcutaneous tissue, and to the anterior chamber of the eye. Br J Exp Pathol 29: 58–69

33. Nicholas MK, Antel JP, Stefanson K, Arnason BGW (1987) Rejection of fetal neocortical neural transplants by H-2 incompatible mice. J Immunol 139: 2275–2283

34. Oluwole SF, Tezuka K, Wasfie T, Stegali MD, Reemtsma K, Hardy MA (1989) Humoral immunity in allograft rejection. The role of cytotoxic antibody in hyperacute rejection and enhancement of rat cardiac allograft. Transplantation 48: 751–755

35. Perry VH, Hume DA, Gordon S (1985) Immunohistochemical localization of macrophages and microglia in the adult and developing mouse brain. Neuroscience 15: 313–326

36. Perry VH, Lund RD (1989) Microglia in retinae transplanted to the central nervous system. Neuroscience 31: 453–462

37. Poltorak M, Freed WJ (1990) Immunological reactions induced by intracerebral transplantation: evidence that host microglia but not astroglia are the antigen-presenting cells. Exp Neurol 103: 222–233

38. Prineas JW (1979) Multiple sclerosis: presence of lymphatic capillaries and lymphoid tissue in the brain and spinal cord. Science 203: 1123–1125

39. Pryce G, Male DK, Sedgwick J (1989) Antigen presentation in the brain: brain endothelial cells are poor simulators of T cell proliferation. Immunology 66: 207–212

40. Sloan DJ, Baker BJ, Puclavec SM, Charlton HM (1990) The effect of site transplantation and histocompatibility differences on the survival of neural tissue transplanted to the CNS of defined inbred strains of rats. Prog Brain Res 82: 141–152

41. Stewart PA, Wiley MJ (1985) Developing nervous tissue induces formation of blood-brain barrier characteristics in invading endothelial cells: a study using quail-chick transplantation chimera. Dev Biol 84: 183–192

42. Svendgaard N-A, Björklund A, Hardebo J-E, Stenevi U (1975) Axonal degeneration associated with a defective blood-brain barrier in cerebral implants. Nature 255: 334–337

43. Traugott U, Scheinberg L, Raine C (1985) On the presence of Ia-positive endothelial cells and astrocytes in multiple sclerosis lesions and its relevance to antigen presentation. J Neuroimmunol 8: 1–14

44. Trotter J, Steinman L (1984) Homing of Lyt-2+ and Lyt-2- T-cell subsets and B lymphocytes to the central nervous system of mice with acute experimental allergic encephalomyelitis. J Immunol 132: 291–293

45. Wekerle H, Linington C, Lassman H, Meyerman R (1986) Cellular immune reactivity within the CNS. Trend Neurosci 9: 271–277

46. Widner H, Brundin P (1988) Immunological aspects of grafting in the mammalian central nervous system. A review and speculative synthesis. Brain Res Rev 13: 287–324

47. Widner H, Brundin P (1993) The effects of a second allogeneic graft on the survival of intracerebral allogeneic fetal neuronal grafts in rats. Cell transplantation (in press)

48. Widner H, Brundin P, Björklund A, Möller E (1989) Survival and immunogenicity of dissociated allogeneic fetal dopaminergic-rich grafts when implanted into the brains of adult mice. Exp Brain Res 76: 187–197

49. Widner H, Möller G, Johansson BB (1988) Immune response in deep cervical lymph nodes and spleen in the mouse after antigen diposition in different intracerebral sites. Scand J Immunol 28: 563–571

50. Widner H, Tetrud J, Rehncrona S, Snow B, Brundin P, Gustavii B, Björklund A, Lindvall O, Langston JW (1992) Bilateral fetal mesencephalic grafting in two patients with parkinsonism induced by 1-methyl-4-phenyl.1, 2, 3, 6- tetrahydropyridine (MPTP). N Engl J Med 327: 1556–1563

51. Yoffey JM, Courtice FC (1970) Lymphatics, lymph and the lymphomyeloid complex. Academic, New York

52. Zhou HF, Lee LH, Lund RD (1990) Timing and patterns of astrocyte migration from xenogeneic transplants of the cortex and corpus callosum. J Comp Neurol 292: 320–330

Basic and Clinical Aspects of Neuroscience

Eds.: **C. Weil, E. E. Müller, M. O. Thorner**

Vol. 4

Somatostatin

With contributions by Y. C. Patel, D. R. Rubinow, C. L. Davis, R. M. Post, V. Schusdziarra, J. Epelbaum, P. N. Maton, R. F. Ayakaki

1992. X, 66 pp. 31 figs. 6 tabs.
ISBN 3-540-54569-7

One of the phylogenetically oldest hormones, somatostatin is a regulatory peptide with remarkable characteristics. It is a nonclassical neurotransmitter discovered less than 20 years ago both in the central nervous system and in the gastroenteropancreatic system. It regulates the secretion of both pituitary and digestive hormones; it ensures nutrient homeostasis and it has therapeutic uses. This volume deals with all these aspects.

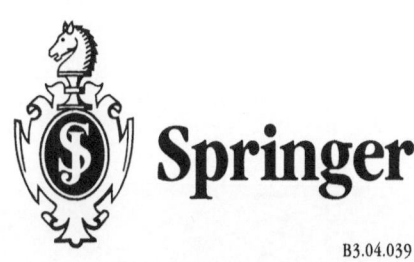

Springer

Basic and Clinical Aspects of Neuroscience

Eds.: **E. Flückiger, E. E. Müller, M. O. Thorner**

Volume 3

The Role of Brain Dopamine

With contributions by P. Riederer, E. Sofic, C. Konradi, J. Kornhuber, H. Beckmann, M. Dietl, G. Moll, G. Hebenstreit, M. O. Thorner, M. L. Vance, J. C. Stoof, F. J. H. Tilders, T. J. Petcher

Cover illustration by J. Haley

1989. 29 figs., 5 tabs. IX, 55 pp. ISBN 3-540-50040-5

As in other volumes in the series, this volume conveys up-to-date knowledge in a clear and straightforward manner. It begins with a survey of the neurobiological functions of the brain, with the emphasis on Parkinson's disease. This is followed by a presentation of the role of dopamine in the regulation of human anterior pituitary function. The final two chapters concentrate on the dopamine receptors: first, the binding sites are characterized and the biochemical and physiological consequences of dopamine-receptor stimulation are discussed and, finally, there is a report on the topology of a dopamine-receptor model that can account comprehensively for agonists and antagonists.

Volume 2

Transmitter Molecules in the Brain

Part 1: Biochemistry of Transmitter Molecules

With contributions by G. Fink, J. McQueen, A. J. Harmar, G. W. Arbuthnott

Part 2: Function and Dysfunction

With contribution by R. Mitchell, J. E. Christie, G. Fink

1987. Out of print.

Volume 1

The Dopaminergic System

With contributions by B. Halasz, K. Fuxe, L. F. Agnati, M. Kalia, M. Goldstein

1985. VIII, 39 pp. 23 figs.
ISBN 3-540-13700-9

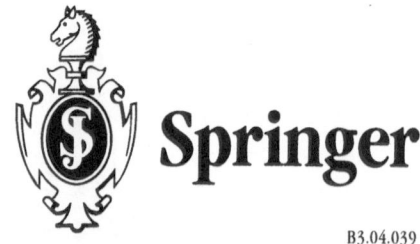

Springer

B3.04.039